Epilepsy Journal for Children

Keep a Log of Your Child's Seizures, Medications, Triggers

& Side Effects

Medjournal Essentials

Epilepsy Journal
Copyright © 2019 by Medjournal Essentials

All rights reserved. No part of this book may be used or reproduced in any manner whatsoever without written permission.

ISBN: 9781796960884

This Journal Belongs To: _____

Emergency Contact

Name:
Relationship:
Telephone:
Mobile:
Address:

Secondary Contact

Name:
Relationship:
Telephone:
Mobile:
Address:

Medical Practitioner

Doctor's Name:
Telephone:
Address:

CONTENTS

INTRODUCTION 1
CALENDAR 3
MEDICATION HISTORY 9
QUESTIONS FOR YOUR DOCTOR 21
SEIZURE LOG 27

Epilepsy Journal

KEEPING A SEIZURE LOG

☙❧

As the parent or caregiver of a child with epilepsy you face many challenges, one of which is keeping track of seizures, medications and side effects. This journal will help you keep that information together in one place. The seizure log pages contain a lot of sections, but you don't have to fill all of them in every time. For example, if you are familiar with the types of seizures your child experiences you may wish to skip the section describing what happens during a seizure, or only use it if something unusual happens. However, if your child is newly diagnosed it may be very helpful to have this information. Discuss with your child's doctor exactly what information they wish you to record.

Why Is It Important to Keep a Seizure Log?

There are several important reasons for keeping a seizure log - to aid in diagnosis, to help you and your doctor to make decisions about treatment, and to help you spot patterns and triggers.

Diagnosis & Treatment Decisions

Writing down what happens before, during and after a seizure can help your doctor identify the type of seizures that your child is experiencing. This is important because some medications are more effective for certain types of seizures. Keeping a record also helps you and your doctor decide whether medications are effective or need changing. If seizures get better, stay the same, or get worse after a medication change everyone needs to know. A log will also help you track side effects from medications that your child takes. All this information helps you and your healthcare provider make informed decisions about treatment. This journal allows you to keep all your notes and questions together and to share them when you take your child to appointments.

Patterns & Triggers

Writing down the time, where your child was and what your child was doing prior to a seizure may help you spot patterns and identify potential triggers. Some common triggers are listed on the seizure record pages as tick box options, and there are spaces to record your own. There is also a notes section for your own observations and thoughts. Identifying triggers could help you find lifestyle changes that may help your child. Keeping records will also help you see if any changes you introduce are making a difference.

Using the Seizure Journal

Seizure Calendar

This journal has a calendar on which you can quickly record the number of seizures on any given day and easily spot frequency over days, weeks and months. You can see how many days have passed between events, or any patterns. More information on using the calendar and an example is included at the beginning of the calendar section.

Medications

Each medication that your child takes has its own page in which you can record the dosage and frequency, record changes and note any side effects.

Questions to Ask Your Doctor

It can be difficult to remember everything you wanted to ask when you are in the consulting room, use this section to note down questions you have for your child's doctor.

Seizure Log

The log pages are written without using medical terms so that family members, schools or care givers can update the journal if needed. Only fill in the information sections that you need, skip any that are not relevant.

One Last Thing

We are always looking to improve, and regularly review our journals to make sure they are meeting your needs. If you have a suggestion for something we can add to future revisions, want to let us know about something we do well, or something we could do better, please get in touch. We read every suggestion we receive and always appreciate your feedback.

Contact us on: customersupport@medjournalessentials.com

Calendar

Using the Seizure Calendar

Use the calendar to record the number of seizures that have happened on any given day. Fill in the year at the top and the current month on the left-hand side (or previous months if you wish to track historical data). If your child only has one type of seizure, write the number in for that day. If your child has several types of seizure, you can give each one a code (a chart is provided below) write the code followed by the number of seizures each day. If there are too many seizures to record on one day, you can write the seizure log page number. If there have been medication or lifestyle changes, you can shade in the relevant days, weeks or months with a coloured pencil allowing you to see if the changes have had an effect. A key is included below.

Month	1	2	3	4	5	6
Jan	F1 T2			P. 32		

Seizure Type	Code	Seizure Type	Code

Colour	Medication / Lifestyle Change

Seizure Calendar   Year: _____

Seizure Calendar

Year:

Seizure Calendar Year: _____

Seizure Calendar

Year:

Medication History

Medication History

Medication & Dose	Date Started	Reason for Starting
	Date Stopped	Reason for Stopping

Changes

Date	New Dose	Reason for Change

Date	Side Effects / Notes

Medication History

Medication & Dose	Date Started	Reason for Starting
	Date Stopped	**Reason for Stopping**

Changes

Date	New Dose	Reason for Change

Date	Side Effects / Notes

Medication History

Medication & Dose	Date Started	Reason for Starting
	Date Stopped	Reason for Stopping

Changes

Date	New Dose	Reason for Change

Date	Side Effects / Notes

Medication History

Medication & Dose	Date Started	Reason for Starting
	Date Stopped	Reason for Stopping

Changes

Date	New Dose	Reason for Change

Date	Side Effects / Notes

Medication History

Medication & Dose	Date Started	Reason for Starting
	Date Stopped	Reason for Stopping

Changes

Date	New Dose	Reason for Change

Date	Side Effects / Notes

Medication History

Medication & Dose	Date Started	Reason for Starting
	Date Stopped	Reason for Stopping

Changes

Date	New Dose	Reason for Change

Date	Side Effects / Notes

Medication History

Medication & Dose	Date Started	Reason for Starting
	Date Stopped	**Reason for Stopping**

Changes

Date	New Dose	Reason for Change

Date	Side Effects / Notes

Medication History

Medication & Dose	Date Started	Reason for Starting
	Date Stopped	**Reason for Stopping**

Changes

Date	New Dose	Reason for Change

Date	Side Effects / Notes

Medication History

Medication & Dose	Date Started	Reason for Starting
	Date Stopped	Reason for Stopping

Changes

Date	New Dose	Reason for Change

Date	Side Effects / Notes

Medication History

Medication & Dose	Date Started	Reason for Starting
	Date Stopped	Reason for Stopping

Changes

Date	New Dose	Reason for Change

Date	Side Effects / Notes

Medication History

Medication & Dose	Date Started	Reason for Starting
	Date Stopped	**Reason for Stopping**

Changes

Date	New Dose	Reason for Change

Date	Side Effects / Notes

Questions to Ask Your Doctor

Questions to Ask Your Doctor

Questions to Ask Your Doctor

Questions to Ask Your Doctor

Questions to Ask Your Doctor

Questions to Ask Your Doctor

Seizure Log

Seizure Log

Date: _____ Time: _____ Duration: _____

Location: _____

Seizure Type: _____

If this was a cluster how many seizures? _____

Child's Mood: _____

What happened during the seizure? _____

_____

_____

_____

What was happening around the time the seizure occurred? _____

_____

_____

Was there an Aura or warning? Yes ☐ No ☐ Describe: _____

_____

Rescue medication if given: _____

VNS applied? Yes ☐ No ☐ Detail: _____

How long did it take your child to recover? _____

Notes: _____

_____

_____

_____

Seizure Log

Possible Triggers			
High temperature		Illness or infection	
Missed or late medication		Temperature change	
Overtired		Missed or Poor Sleep	
Mood Change		Fast Breathing	
Missed Meal		Specific Food	
During Sleep		Upon Waking	
Time of day		Screen Use	
Low blood sugar		Low blood sodium	
OTC medications or supplements (please list)		Exercise (What did your child do?)	
Strong emotions - anxiety, stress, excitement, anger. Please describe:		Sensory - sounds, bright colours, flashing lights, patterns. Please describe:	
Other:		Other:	
Other:		Other:	

What happened after? (Recovery Period)			
Muscle weakness		Blurred or double vision	
Speech changes		Confusion	
Tired or sleepy		Remembers the event	
Shaking / tremors		Feeling light-headed	
Problems communicating		Unsteady walking	
Loss of coordination (clumsy)		Change in appetite	
Digestive problems		Nausea / Vomiting	
Change in mood: depression, agitation, anger, irritability, excitability		Numbness (name part of body)	
Change in behaviour (detail in notes)		Headache	
Other:		Other:	
Other:		Other:	

Seizure Log

Date: Time: Duration:

Location:

Seizure Type:

If this was a cluster how many seizures?

Child's Mood:

What happened during the seizure?

What was happening around the time the seizure occurred?

Was there an Aura or warning? Yes ☐ No ☐ Describe:

Rescue medication if given:

VNS applied? Yes ☐ No ☐ Detail:

How long did it take your child to recover?

Notes:

Seizure Log

Possible Triggers

High temperature		Illness or infection	
Missed or late medication		Temperature change	
Overtired		Missed or Poor Sleep	
Mood Change		Fast Breathing	
Missed Meal		Specific Food	
During Sleep		Upon Waking	
Time of day		Screen Use	
Low blood sugar		Low blood sodium	
OTC medications or supplements (please list)		Exercise (What did your child do?)	
Strong emotions - anxiety, stress, excitement, anger. Please describe:		Sensory - sounds, bright colours, flashing lights, patterns. Please describe:	
Other:		Other:	
Other:		Other:	

What happened after? (Recovery Period)

Muscle weakness		Blurred or double vision	
Speech changes		Confusion	
Tired or sleepy		Remembers the event	
Shaking / tremors		Feeling light-headed	
Problems communicating		Unsteady walking	
Loss of coordination (clumsy)		Change in appetite	
Digestive problems		Nausea / Vomiting	
Change in mood: depression, agitation, anger, irritability, excitability		Numbness (name part of body)	
Change in behaviour (detail in notes)		Headache	
Other:		Other:	
Other:		Other:	

Seizure Log

Date: _____ Time: _____ Duration: _____

Location: _____

Seizure Type: _____

If this was a cluster how many seizures? _____

Child's Mood: _____

What happened during the seizure? _____

_____

_____

_____

What was happening around the time the seizure occurred? _____

_____

_____

Was there an Aura or warning? Yes ☐ No ☐ Describe: _____

_____

Rescue medication if given: _____

VNS applied? Yes ☐ No ☐ Detail: _____

How long did it take your child to recover? _____

Notes: _____

_____

_____

_____

Seizure Log

Possible Triggers			
High temperature		Illness or infection	
Missed or late medication		Temperature change	
Overtired		Missed or Poor Sleep	
Mood Change		Fast Breathing	
Missed Meal		Specific Food	
During Sleep		Upon Waking	
Time of day		Screen Use	
Low blood sugar		Low blood sodium	
OTC medications or supplements (please list)		Exercise (What did your child do?)	
Strong emotions - anxiety, stress, excitement, anger. Please describe:		Sensory - sounds, bright colours, flashing lights, patterns. Please describe:	
Other:		Other:	
Other:		Other:	

What happened after? (Recovery Period)			
Muscle weakness		Blurred or double vision	
Speech changes		Confusion	
Tired or sleepy		Remembers the event	
Shaking / tremors		Feeling light-headed	
Problems communicating		Unsteady walking	
Loss of coordination (clumsy)		Change in appetite	
Digestive problems		Nausea / Vomiting	
Change in mood: depression, agitation, anger, irritability, excitability		Numbness (name part of body)	
Change in behaviour (detail in notes)		Headache	
Other:		Other:	
Other:		Other:	

Seizure Log

Date: Time: Duration:

Location:

Seizure Type:

If this was a cluster how many seizures?

Child's Mood:

What happened during the seizure?

What was happening around the time the seizure occurred?

Was there an Aura or warning? Yes ☐ No ☐ Describe:

Rescue medication if given:

VNS applied? Yes ☐ No ☐ Detail:

How long did it take your child to recover?

Notes:

Seizure Log

Possible Triggers			
High temperature		Illness or infection	
Missed or late medication		Temperature change	
Overtired		Missed or Poor Sleep	
Mood Change		Fast Breathing	
Missed Meal		Specific Food	
During Sleep		Upon Waking	
Time of day		Screen Use	
Low blood sugar		Low blood sodium	
OTC medications or supplements (please list)		Exercise (What did your child do?)	
Strong emotions - anxiety, stress, excitement, anger. Please describe:		Sensory - sounds, bright colours, flashing lights, patterns. Please describe:	
Other:		Other:	
Other:		Other:	

What happened after? (Recovery Period)			
Muscle weakness		Blurred or double vision	
Speech changes		Confusion	
Tired or sleepy		Remembers the event	
Shaking / tremors		Feeling light-headed	
Problems communicating		Unsteady walking	
Loss of coordination (clumsy)		Change in appetite	
Digestive problems		Nausea / Vomiting	
Change in mood: depression, agitation, anger, irritability, excitability		Numbness (name part of body)	
Change in behaviour (detail in notes)		Headache	
Other:		Other:	
Other:		Other:	

Seizure Log

Date: Time: Duration:

Location:

Seizure Type:

If this was a cluster how many seizures?

Child's Mood:

What happened during the seizure?

What was happening around the time the seizure occurred?

Was there an Aura or warning? Yes ☐   No ☐   Describe:

Rescue medication if given:

VNS applied? Yes ☐   No ☐   Detail:

How long did it take your child to recover?

Notes:

Seizure Log

Possible Triggers			
High temperature		Illness or infection	
Missed or late medication		Temperature change	
Overtired		Missed or Poor Sleep	
Mood Change		Fast Breathing	
Missed Meal		Specific Food	
During Sleep		Upon Waking	
Time of day		Screen Use	
Low blood sugar		Low blood sodium	
OTC medications or supplements (please list)		Exercise (What did your child do?)	
Strong emotions - anxiety, stress, excitement, anger. Please describe:		Sensory - sounds, bright colours, flashing lights, patterns. Please describe:	
Other:		Other:	
Other:		Other:	

What happened after? (Recovery Period)			
Muscle weakness		Blurred or double vision	
Speech changes		Confusion	
Tired or sleepy		Remembers the event	
Shaking / tremors		Feeling light-headed	
Problems communicating		Unsteady walking	
Loss of coordination (clumsy)		Change in appetite	
Digestive problems		Nausea / Vomiting	
Change in mood: depression, agitation, anger, irritability, excitability		Numbness (name part of body)	
Change in behaviour (detail in notes)		Headache	
Other:		Other:	
Other:		Other:	

Seizure Log

Date: _____ Time: _____ Duration: _____

Location:

Seizure Type:

If this was a cluster how many seizures?

Child's Mood:

What happened during the seizure?

What was happening around the time the seizure occurred?

Was there an Aura or warning? Yes ☐ No ☐ Describe:

Rescue medication if given:

VNS applied? Yes ☐ No ☐ Detail:

How long did it take your child to recover?

Notes:

Seizure Log

Possible Triggers			
High temperature		Illness or infection	
Missed or late medication		Temperature change	
Overtired		Missed or Poor Sleep	
Mood Change		Fast Breathing	
Missed Meal		Specific Food	
During Sleep		Upon Waking	
Time of day		Screen Use	
Low blood sugar		Low blood sodium	
OTC medications or supplements (please list)		Exercise (What did your child do?)	
Strong emotions - anxiety, stress, excitement, anger. Please describe:		Sensory - sounds, bright colours, flashing lights, patterns. Please describe:	
Other:		Other:	
Other:		Other:	

What happened after? (Recovery Period)			
Muscle weakness		Blurred or double vision	
Speech changes		Confusion	
Tired or sleepy		Remembers the event	
Shaking / tremors		Feeling light-headed	
Problems communicating		Unsteady walking	
Loss of coordination (clumsy)		Change in appetite	
Digestive problems		Nausea / Vomiting	
Change in mood: depression, agitation, anger, irritability, excitability		Numbness (name part of body)	
Change in behaviour (detail in notes)		Headache	
Other:		Other:	
Other:		Other:	

Seizure Log

Date: Time: Duration:

Location:

Seizure Type:

If this was a cluster how many seizures?

Child's Mood:

What happened during the seizure?

What was happening around the time the seizure occurred?

Was there an Aura or warning? Yes ☐ No ☐ Describe:

Rescue medication if given:

VNS applied? Yes ☐ No ☐ Detail:

How long did it take your child to recover?

Notes:

Seizure Log

Possible Triggers

High temperature		Illness or infection	
Missed or late medication		Temperature change	
Overtired		Missed or Poor Sleep	
Mood Change		Fast Breathing	
Missed Meal		Specific Food	
During Sleep		Upon Waking	
Time of day		Screen Use	
Low blood sugar		Low blood sodium	
OTC medications or supplements (please list)		Exercise (What did your child do?)	
Strong emotions - anxiety, stress, excitement, anger. Please describe:		Sensory - sounds, bright colours, flashing lights, patterns. Please describe:	
Other:		Other:	
Other:		Other:	

What happened after? (Recovery Period)

Muscle weakness		Blurred or double vision	
Speech changes		Confusion	
Tired or sleepy		Remembers the event	
Shaking / tremors		Feeling light-headed	
Problems communicating		Unsteady walking	
Loss of coordination (clumsy)		Change in appetite	
Digestive problems		Nausea / Vomiting	
Change in mood: depression, agitation, anger, irritability, excitability		Numbness (name part of body)	
Change in behaviour (detail in notes)		Headache	
Other:		Other:	
Other:		Other:	

Seizure Log

Date: Time: Duration:

Location:

Seizure Type:

If this was a cluster how many seizures?

Child's Mood:

What happened during the seizure?

What was happening around the time the seizure occurred?

Was there an Aura or warning? Yes ☐ No ☐ Describe:

Rescue medication if given:

VNS applied? Yes ☐ No ☐ Detail:

How long did it take your child to recover?

Notes:

Seizure Log

Possible Triggers

High temperature		Illness or infection	
Missed or late medication		Temperature change	
Overtired		Missed or Poor Sleep	
Mood Change		Fast Breathing	
Missed Meal		Specific Food	
During Sleep		Upon Waking	
Time of day		Screen Use	
Low blood sugar		Low blood sodium	
OTC medications or supplements (please list)		Exercise (What did your child do?)	
Strong emotions - anxiety, stress, excitement, anger. Please describe:		Sensory - sounds, bright colours, flashing lights, patterns. Please describe:	
Other:		Other:	
Other:		Other:	

What happened after? (Recovery Period)

Muscle weakness		Blurred or double vision	
Speech changes		Confusion	
Tired or sleepy		Remembers the event	
Shaking / tremors		Feeling light-headed	
Problems communicating		Unsteady walking	
Loss of coordination (clumsy)		Change in appetite	
Digestive problems		Nausea / Vomiting	
Change in mood: depression, agitation, anger, irritability, excitability		Numbness (name part of body)	
Change in behaviour (detail in notes)		Headache	
Other:		Other:	
Other:		Other:	

Seizure Log

Date: _____ Time: _____ Duration: _____

Location: _____

Seizure Type: _____

If this was a cluster how many seizures? _____

Child's Mood: _____

What happened during the seizure? _____

_____

_____

_____

What was happening around the time the seizure occurred? _____

_____

_____

_____

Was there an Aura or warning? Yes ☐ No ☐ Describe: _____

_____

Rescue medication if given: _____

VNS applied? Yes ☐ No ☐ Detail: _____

How long did it take your child to recover? _____

Notes: _____

_____

_____

_____

_____

Seizure Log

Possible Triggers			
High temperature		Illness or infection	
Missed or late medication		Temperature change	
Overtired		Missed or Poor Sleep	
Mood Change		Fast Breathing	
Missed Meal		Specific Food	
During Sleep		Upon Waking	
Time of day		Screen Use	
Low blood sugar		Low blood sodium	
OTC medications or supplements (please list)		Exercise (What did your child do?)	
Strong emotions - anxiety, stress, excitement, anger. Please describe:		Sensory - sounds, bright colours, flashing lights, patterns. Please describe:	
Other:		Other:	
Other:		Other:	

What happened after? (Recovery Period)			
Muscle weakness		Blurred or double vision	
Speech changes		Confusion	
Tired or sleepy		Remembers the event	
Shaking / tremors		Feeling light-headed	
Problems communicating		Unsteady walking	
Loss of coordination (clumsy)		Change in appetite	
Digestive problems		Nausea / Vomiting	
Change in mood: depression, agitation, anger, irritability, excitability		Numbness (name part of body)	
Change in behaviour (detail in notes)		Headache	
Other:		Other:	
Other:		Other:	

Seizure Log

Date: Time: Duration:

Location:

Seizure Type:

If this was a cluster how many seizures?

Child's Mood:

What happened during the seizure?

What was happening around the time the seizure occurred?

Was there an Aura or warning? Yes ☐ No ☐ Describe:

Rescue medication if given:

VNS applied? Yes ☐ No ☐ Detail:

How long did it take your child to recover?

Notes:

Seizure Log

Possible Triggers			
High temperature		Illness or infection	
Missed or late medication		Temperature change	
Overtired		Missed or Poor Sleep	
Mood Change		Fast Breathing	
Missed Meal		Specific Food	
During Sleep		Upon Waking	
Time of day		Screen Use	
Low blood sugar		Low blood sodium	
OTC medications or supplements (please list)		Exercise (What did your child do?)	
Strong emotions - anxiety, stress, excitement, anger. Please describe:		Sensory - sounds, bright colours, flashing lights, patterns. Please describe:	
Other:		Other:	
Other:		Other:	

What happened after? (Recovery Period)			
Muscle weakness		Blurred or double vision	
Speech changes		Confusion	
Tired or sleepy		Remembers the event	
Shaking / tremors		Feeling light-headed	
Problems communicating		Unsteady walking	
Loss of coordination (clumsy)		Change in appetite	
Digestive problems		Nausea / Vomiting	
Change in mood: depression, agitation, anger, irritability, excitability		Numbness (name part of body)	
Change in behaviour (detail in notes)		Headache	
Other:		Other:	
Other:		Other:	

Seizure Log

Date: Time: Duration:

Location:

Seizure Type:

If this was a cluster how many seizures?

Child's Mood:

What happened during the seizure?

What was happening around the time the seizure occurred?

Was there an Aura or warning? Yes ☐ No ☐ Describe:

Rescue medication if given:

VNS applied? Yes ☐ No ☐ Detail:

How long did it take your child to recover?

Notes:

Seizure Log

Possible Triggers			
High temperature		Illness or infection	
Missed or late medication		Temperature change	
Overtired		Missed or Poor Sleep	
Mood Change		Fast Breathing	
Missed Meal		Specific Food	
During Sleep		Upon Waking	
Time of day		Screen Use	
Low blood sugar		Low blood sodium	
OTC medications or supplements (please list)		Exercise (What did your child do?)	
Strong emotions - anxiety, stress, excitement, anger. Please describe:		Sensory - sounds, bright colours, flashing lights, patterns. Please describe:	
Other:		Other:	
Other:		Other:	

What happened after? (Recovery Period)			
Muscle weakness		Blurred or double vision	
Speech changes		Confusion	
Tired or sleepy		Remembers the event	
Shaking / tremors		Feeling light-headed	
Problems communicating		Unsteady walking	
Loss of coordination (clumsy)		Change in appetite	
Digestive problems		Nausea / Vomiting	
Change in mood: depression, agitation, anger, irritability, excitability		Numbness (name part of body)	
Change in behaviour (detail in notes)		Headache	
Other:		Other:	
Other:		Other:	

Seizure Log

Date: Time: Duration:

Location:

Seizure Type:

If this was a cluster how many seizures?

Child's Mood:

What happened during the seizure?

What was happening around the time the seizure occurred?

Was there an Aura or warning? Yes ☐ No ☐ Describe:

Rescue medication if given:

VNS applied? Yes ☐ No ☐ Detail:

How long did it take your child to recover?

Notes:

Seizure Log

Possible Triggers			
High temperature		Illness or infection	
Missed or late medication		Temperature change	
Overtired		Missed or Poor Sleep	
Mood Change		Fast Breathing	
Missed Meal		Specific Food	
During Sleep		Upon Waking	
Time of day		Screen Use	
Low blood sugar		Low blood sodium	
OTC medications or supplements (please list)		Exercise (What did your child do?)	
Strong emotions - anxiety, stress, excitement, anger. Please describe:		Sensory - sounds, bright colours, flashing lights, patterns. Please describe:	
Other:		Other:	
Other:		Other:	

What happened after? (Recovery Period)			
Muscle weakness		Blurred or double vision	
Speech changes		Confusion	
Tired or sleepy		Remembers the event	
Shaking / tremors		Feeling light-headed	
Problems communicating		Unsteady walking	
Loss of coordination (clumsy)		Change in appetite	
Digestive problems		Nausea / Vomiting	
Change in mood: depression, agitation, anger, irritability, excitability		Numbness (name part of body)	
Change in behaviour (detail in notes)		Headache	
Other:		Other:	
Other:		Other:	

Seizure Log

Date: Time: Duration:

Location:

Seizure Type:

If this was a cluster how many seizures?

Child's Mood:

What happened during the seizure?

What was happening around the time the seizure occurred?

Was there an Aura or warning?   Yes ☐   No ☐   Describe:

Rescue medication if given:

VNS applied? Yes ☐   No ☐   Detail:

How long did it take your child to recover?

Notes:

Seizure Log

Possible Triggers

High temperature		Illness or infection	
Missed or late medication		Temperature change	
Overtired		Missed or Poor Sleep	
Mood Change		Fast Breathing	
Missed Meal		Specific Food	
During Sleep		Upon Waking	
Time of day		Screen Use	
Low blood sugar		Low blood sodium	
OTC medications or supplements (please list)		Exercise (What did your child do?)	
Strong emotions - anxiety, stress, excitement, anger. Please describe:		Sensory - sounds, bright colours, flashing lights, patterns. Please describe:	
Other:		Other:	
Other:		Other:	

What happened after? (Recovery Period)

Muscle weakness		Blurred or double vision	
Speech changes		Confusion	
Tired or sleepy		Remembers the event	
Shaking / tremors		Feeling light-headed	
Problems communicating		Unsteady walking	
Loss of coordination (clumsy)		Change in appetite	
Digestive problems		Nausea / Vomiting	
Change in mood: depression, agitation, anger, irritability, excitability		Numbness (name part of body)	
Change in behaviour (detail in notes)		Headache	
Other:		Other:	
Other:		Other:	

Seizure Log

Date: _____ Time: _____ Duration: _____

Location: _____

Seizure Type: _____

If this was a cluster how many seizures? _____

Child's Mood: _____

What happened during the seizure?
_____
_____
_____
_____

What was happening around the time the seizure occurred?
_____
_____
_____

Was there an Aura or warning? Yes ☐ No ☐ Describe: _____
_____

Rescue medication if given: _____

VNS applied? Yes ☐ No ☐ Detail: _____

How long did it take your child to recover? _____

Notes:
_____
_____
_____
_____

Seizure Log

Possible Triggers			
High temperature		Illness or infection	
Missed or late medication		Temperature change	
Overtired		Missed or Poor Sleep	
Mood Change		Fast Breathing	
Missed Meal		Specific Food	
During Sleep		Upon Waking	
Time of day		Screen Use	
Low blood sugar		Low blood sodium	
OTC medications or supplements (please list)		Exercise (What did your child do?)	
Strong emotions - anxiety, stress, excitement, anger. Please describe:		Sensory - sounds, bright colours, flashing lights, patterns. Please describe:	
Other:		Other:	
Other:		Other:	

What happened after? (Recovery Period)			
Muscle weakness		Blurred or double vision	
Speech changes		Confusion	
Tired or sleepy		Remembers the event	
Shaking / tremors		Feeling light-headed	
Problems communicating		Unsteady walking	
Loss of coordination (clumsy)		Change in appetite	
Digestive problems		Nausea / Vomiting	
Change in mood: depression, agitation, anger, irritability, excitability		Numbness (name part of body)	
Change in behaviour (detail in notes)		Headache	
Other:		Other:	
Other:		Other:	

Seizure Log

Date: Time: Duration:

Location:

Seizure Type:

If this was a cluster how many seizures?

Child's Mood:

What happened during the seizure?

What was happening around the time the seizure occurred?

Was there an Aura or warning? Yes ☐ No ☐ Describe:

Rescue medication if given:

VNS applied? Yes ☐ No ☐ Detail:

How long did it take your child to recover?

Notes:

Seizure Log

Possible Triggers

High temperature	Illness or infection
Missed or late medication	Temperature change
Overtired	Missed or Poor Sleep
Mood Change	Fast Breathing
Missed Meal	Specific Food
During Sleep	Upon Waking
Time of day	Screen Use
Low blood sugar	Low blood sodium
OTC medications or supplements (please list)	Exercise (What did your child do?)
Strong emotions - anxiety, stress, excitement, anger. Please describe:	Sensory - sounds, bright colours, flashing lights, patterns. Please describe:
Other:	Other:
Other:	Other:

What happened after? (Recovery Period)

Muscle weakness	Blurred or double vision
Speech changes	Confusion
Tired or sleepy	Remembers the event
Shaking / tremors	Feeling light-headed
Problems communicating	Unsteady walking
Loss of coordination (clumsy)	Change in appetite
Digestive problems	Nausea / Vomiting
Change in mood: depression, agitation, anger, irritability, excitability	Numbness (name part of body)
Change in behaviour (detail in notes)	Headache
Other:	Other:
Other:	Other:

Seizure Log

Date: Time: Duration:

Location:

Seizure Type:

If this was a cluster how many seizures?

Child's Mood:

What happened during the seizure?

What was happening around the time the seizure occurred?

Was there an Aura or warning? Yes ☐ No ☐ Describe:

Rescue medication if given:

VNS applied? Yes ☐ No ☐ Detail:

How long did it take your child to recover?

Notes:

Seizure Log

Possible Triggers

High temperature		Illness or infection	
Missed or late medication		Temperature change	
Overtired		Missed or Poor Sleep	
Mood Change		Fast Breathing	
Missed Meal		Specific Food	
During Sleep		Upon Waking	
Time of day		Screen Use	
Low blood sugar		Low blood sodium	
OTC medications or supplements (please list)		Exercise (What did your child do?)	
Strong emotions - anxiety, stress, excitement, anger. Please describe:		Sensory - sounds, bright colours, flashing lights, patterns. Please describe:	
Other:		Other:	
Other:		Other:	

What happened after? (Recovery Period)

Muscle weakness		Blurred or double vision	
Speech changes		Confusion	
Tired or sleepy		Remembers the event	
Shaking / tremors		Feeling light-headed	
Problems communicating		Unsteady walking	
Loss of coordination (clumsy)		Change in appetite	
Digestive problems		Nausea / Vomiting	
Change in mood: depression, agitation, anger, irritability, excitability		Numbness (name part of body)	
Change in behaviour (detail in notes)		Headache	
Other:		Other:	
Other:		Other:	

Seizure Log

Date:	Time:	Duration:

Location:

Seizure Type:

If this was a cluster how many seizures?

Child's Mood:

What happened during the seizure?

What was happening around the time the seizure occurred?

Was there an Aura or warning? Yes ☐ No ☐ Describe:

Rescue medication if given:

VNS applied? Yes ☐ No ☐ Detail:

How long did it take your child to recover?

Notes:

Seizure Log

Possible Triggers			
High temperature		Illness or infection	
Missed or late medication		Temperature change	
Overtired		Missed or Poor Sleep	
Mood Change		Fast Breathing	
Missed Meal		Specific Food	
During Sleep		Upon Waking	
Time of day		Screen Use	
Low blood sugar		Low blood sodium	
OTC medications or supplements (please list)		Exercise (What did your child do?)	
Strong emotions - anxiety, stress, excitement, anger. Please describe:		Sensory - sounds, bright colours, flashing lights, patterns. Please describe:	
Other:		Other:	
Other:		Other:	

What happened after? (Recovery Period)			
Muscle weakness		Blurred or double vision	
Speech changes		Confusion	
Tired or sleepy		Remembers the event	
Shaking / tremors		Feeling light-headed	
Problems communicating		Unsteady walking	
Loss of coordination (clumsy)		Change in appetite	
Digestive problems		Nausea / Vomiting	
Change in mood: depression, agitation, anger, irritability, excitability		Numbness (name part of body)	
Change in behaviour (detail in notes)		Headache	
Other:		Other:	
Other:		Other:	

Seizure Log

Date: Time: Duration:

Location:

Seizure Type:

If this was a cluster how many seizures?

Child's Mood:

What happened during the seizure?

What was happening around the time the seizure occurred?

Was there an Aura or warning? Yes ☐ No ☐ Describe:

Rescue medication if given:

VNS applied? Yes ☐ No ☐ Detail:

How long did it take your child to recover?

Notes:

Seizure Log

Possible Triggers			
High temperature		Illness or infection	
Missed or late medication		Temperature change	
Overtired		Missed or Poor Sleep	
Mood Change		Fast Breathing	
Missed Meal		Specific Food	
During Sleep		Upon Waking	
Time of day		Screen Use	
Low blood sugar		Low blood sodium	
OTC medications or supplements (please list)		Exercise (What did your child do?)	
Strong emotions - anxiety, stress, excitement, anger. Please describe:		Sensory - sounds, bright colours, flashing lights, patterns. Please describe:	
Other:		Other:	
Other:		Other:	

What happened after? (Recovery Period)			
Muscle weakness		Blurred or double vision	
Speech changes		Confusion	
Tired or sleepy		Remembers the event	
Shaking / tremors		Feeling light-headed	
Problems communicating		Unsteady walking	
Loss of coordination (clumsy)		Change in appetite	
Digestive problems		Nausea / Vomiting	
Change in mood: depression, agitation, anger, irritability, excitability		Numbness (name part of body)	
Change in behaviour (detail in notes)		Headache	
Other:		Other:	
Other:		Other:	

Seizure Log

Date: Time: Duration:

Location:

Seizure Type:

If this was a cluster how many seizures?

Child's Mood:

What happened during the seizure?

What was happening around the time the seizure occurred?

Was there an Aura or warning?   Yes ☐   No ☐   Describe:

Rescue medication if given:

VNS applied? Yes ☐   No ☐   Detail:

How long did it take your child to recover?

Notes:

Seizure Log

Possible Triggers			
High temperature		Illness or infection	
Missed or late medication		Temperature change	
Overtired		Missed or Poor Sleep	
Mood Change		Fast Breathing	
Missed Meal		Specific Food	
During Sleep		Upon Waking	
Time of day		Screen Use	
Low blood sugar		Low blood sodium	
OTC medications or supplements (please list)		Exercise (What did your child do?)	
Strong emotions - anxiety, stress, excitement, anger. Please describe:		Sensory - sounds, bright colours, flashing lights, patterns. Please describe:	
Other:		Other:	
Other:		Other:	

What happened after? (Recovery Period)			
Muscle weakness		Blurred or double vision	
Speech changes		Confusion	
Tired or sleepy		Remembers the event	
Shaking / tremors		Feeling light-headed	
Problems communicating		Unsteady walking	
Loss of coordination (clumsy)		Change in appetite	
Digestive problems		Nausea / Vomiting	
Change in mood: depression, agitation, anger, irritability, excitability		Numbness (name part of body)	
Change in behaviour (detail in notes)		Headache	
Other:		Other:	
Other:		Other:	

Seizure Log

Date: Time: Duration:

Location:

Seizure Type:

If this was a cluster how many seizures?

Child's Mood:

What happened during the seizure?

What was happening around the time the seizure occurred?

Was there an Aura or warning? Yes ☐ No ☐ Describe:

Rescue medication if given:

VNS applied? Yes ☐ No ☐ Detail:

How long did it take your child to recover?

Notes:

Seizure Log

Possible Triggers			
High temperature		Illness or infection	
Missed or late medication		Temperature change	
Overtired		Missed or Poor Sleep	
Mood Change		Fast Breathing	
Missed Meal		Specific Food	
During Sleep		Upon Waking	
Time of day		Screen Use	
Low blood sugar		Low blood sodium	
OTC medications or supplements (please list)		Exercise (What did your child do?)	
Strong emotions - anxiety, stress, excitement, anger. Please describe:		Sensory - sounds, bright colours, flashing lights, patterns. Please describe:	
Other:		Other:	
Other:		Other:	

What happened after? (Recovery Period)			
Muscle weakness		Blurred or double vision	
Speech changes		Confusion	
Tired or sleepy		Remembers the event	
Shaking / tremors		Feeling light-headed	
Problems communicating		Unsteady walking	
Loss of coordination (clumsy)		Change in appetite	
Digestive problems		Nausea / Vomiting	
Change in mood: depression, agitation, anger, irritability, excitability		Numbness (name part of body)	
Change in behaviour (detail in notes)		Headache	
Other:		Other:	
Other:		Other:	

Seizure Log

Date: Time: Duration:

Location:

Seizure Type:

If this was a cluster how many seizures?

Child's Mood:

What happened during the seizure?

What was happening around the time the seizure occurred?

Was there an Aura or warning?   Yes ☐   No ☐   Describe:

Rescue medication if given:

VNS applied? Yes ☐   No ☐   Detail:

How long did it take your child to recover?

Notes:

Seizure Log

Possible Triggers			
High temperature		Illness or infection	
Missed or late medication		Temperature change	
Overtired		Missed or Poor Sleep	
Mood Change		Fast Breathing	
Missed Meal		Specific Food	
During Sleep		Upon Waking	
Time of day		Screen Use	
Low blood sugar		Low blood sodium	
OTC medications or supplements (please list)		Exercise (What did your child do?)	
Strong emotions - anxiety, stress, excitement, anger. Please describe:		Sensory - sounds, bright colours, flashing lights, patterns. Please describe:	
Other:		Other:	
Other:		Other:	

What happened after? (Recovery Period)			
Muscle weakness		Blurred or double vision	
Speech changes		Confusion	
Tired or sleepy		Remembers the event	
Shaking / tremors		Feeling light-headed	
Problems communicating		Unsteady walking	
Loss of coordination (clumsy)		Change in appetite	
Digestive problems		Nausea / Vomiting	
Change in mood: depression, agitation, anger, irritability, excitability		Numbness (name part of body)	
Change in behaviour (detail in notes)		Headache	
Other:		Other:	
Other:		Other:	

Seizure Log

Date: Time: Duration:

Location:

Seizure Type:

If this was a cluster how many seizures?

Child's Mood:

What happened during the seizure?

What was happening around the time the seizure occurred?

Was there an Aura or warning? Yes ☐ No ☐ Describe:

Rescue medication if given:

VNS applied? Yes ☐ No ☐ Detail:

How long did it take your child to recover?

Notes:

Seizure Log

Possible Triggers			
High temperature		Illness or infection	
Missed or late medication		Temperature change	
Overtired		Missed or Poor Sleep	
Mood Change		Fast Breathing	
Missed Meal		Specific Food	
During Sleep		Upon Waking	
Time of day		Screen Use	
Low blood sugar		Low blood sodium	
OTC medications or supplements (please list)		Exercise (What did your child do?)	
Strong emotions - anxiety, stress, excitement, anger. Please describe:		Sensory - sounds, bright colours, flashing lights, patterns. Please describe:	
Other:		Other:	
Other:		Other:	

What happened after? (Recovery Period)			
Muscle weakness		Blurred or double vision	
Speech changes		Confusion	
Tired or sleepy		Remembers the event	
Shaking / tremors		Feeling light-headed	
Problems communicating		Unsteady walking	
Loss of coordination (clumsy)		Change in appetite	
Digestive problems		Nausea / Vomiting	
Change in mood: depression, agitation, anger, irritability, excitability		Numbness (name part of body)	
Change in behaviour (detail in notes)		Headache	
Other:		Other:	
Other:		Other:	

Seizure Log

Date: Time: Duration:

Location:

Seizure Type:

If this was a cluster how many seizures?

Child's Mood:

What happened during the seizure?

What was happening around the time the seizure occurred?

Was there an Aura or warning? Yes ☐ No ☐ Describe:

Rescue medication if given:

VNS applied? Yes ☐ No ☐ Detail:

How long did it take your child to recover?

Notes:

Seizure Log

Possible Triggers			
High temperature		Illness or infection	
Missed or late medication		Temperature change	
Overtired		Missed or Poor Sleep	
Mood Change		Fast Breathing	
Missed Meal		Specific Food	
During Sleep		Upon Waking	
Time of day		Screen Use	
Low blood sugar		Low blood sodium	
OTC medications or supplements (please list)		Exercise (What did your child do?)	
Strong emotions - anxiety, stress, excitement, anger. Please describe:		Sensory - sounds, bright colours, flashing lights, patterns. Please describe:	
Other:		Other:	
Other:		Other:	

What happened after? (Recovery Period)			
Muscle weakness		Blurred or double vision	
Speech changes		Confusion	
Tired or sleepy		Remembers the event	
Shaking / tremors		Feeling light-headed	
Problems communicating		Unsteady walking	
Loss of coordination (clumsy)		Change in appetite	
Digestive problems		Nausea / Vomiting	
Change in mood: depression, agitation, anger, irritability, excitability		Numbness (name part of body)	
Change in behaviour (detail in notes)		Headache	
Other:		Other:	
Other:		Other:	

Seizure Log

Date: _____ Time: _____ Duration: _____

Location: _____

Seizure Type: _____

If this was a cluster how many seizures? _____

Child's Mood: _____

What happened during the seizure? _____

What was happening around the time the seizure occurred? _____

Was there an Aura or warning? Yes ☐ No ☐ Describe: _____

Rescue medication if given: _____

VNS applied? Yes ☐ No ☐ Detail: _____

How long did it take your child to recover? _____

Notes: _____

Seizure Log

Possible Triggers			
High temperature		Illness or infection	
Missed or late medication		Temperature change	
Overtired		Missed or Poor Sleep	
Mood Change		Fast Breathing	
Missed Meal		Specific Food	
During Sleep		Upon Waking	
Time of day		Screen Use	
Low blood sugar		Low blood sodium	
OTC medications or supplements (please list)		Exercise (What did your child do?)	
Strong emotions - anxiety, stress, excitement, anger. Please describe:		Sensory - sounds, bright colours, flashing lights, patterns. Please describe:	
Other:		Other:	
Other:		Other:	

What happened after? (Recovery Period)			
Muscle weakness		Blurred or double vision	
Speech changes		Confusion	
Tired or sleepy		Remembers the event	
Shaking / tremors		Feeling light-headed	
Problems communicating		Unsteady walking	
Loss of coordination (clumsy)		Change in appetite	
Digestive problems		Nausea / Vomiting	
Change in mood: depression, agitation, anger, irritability, excitability		Numbness (name part of body)	
Change in behaviour (detail in notes)		Headache	
Other:		Other:	
Other:		Other:	

Seizure Log

Date: Time: Duration:

Location:

Seizure Type:

If this was a cluster how many seizures?

Child's Mood:

What happened during the seizure?

What was happening around the time the seizure occurred?

Was there an Aura or warning? Yes ☐ No ☐ Describe:

Rescue medication if given:

VNS applied? Yes ☐ No ☐ Detail:

How long did it take your child to recover?

Notes:

Seizure Log

Possible Triggers			
High temperature		Illness or infection	
Missed or late medication		Temperature change	
Overtired		Missed or Poor Sleep	
Mood Change		Fast Breathing	
Missed Meal		Specific Food	
During Sleep		Upon Waking	
Time of day		Screen Use	
Low blood sugar		Low blood sodium	
OTC medications or supplements (please list)		Exercise (What did your child do?)	
Strong emotions - anxiety, stress, excitement, anger. Please describe:		Sensory - sounds, bright colours, flashing lights, patterns. Please describe:	
Other:		Other:	
Other:		Other:	

What happened after? (Recovery Period)			
Muscle weakness		Blurred or double vision	
Speech changes		Confusion	
Tired or sleepy		Remembers the event	
Shaking / tremors		Feeling light-headed	
Problems communicating		Unsteady walking	
Loss of coordination (clumsy)		Change in appetite	
Digestive problems		Nausea / Vomiting	
Change in mood: depression, agitation, anger, irritability, excitability		Numbness (name part of body)	
Change in behaviour (detail in notes)		Headache	
Other:		Other:	
Other:		Other:	

Seizure Log

Date: Time: Duration:

Location:

Seizure Type:

If this was a cluster how many seizures?

Child's Mood:

What happened during the seizure?

What was happening around the time the seizure occurred?

Was there an Aura or warning? Yes ☐ No ☐ Describe:

Rescue medication if given:

VNS applied? Yes ☐ No ☐ Detail:

How long did it take your child to recover?

Notes:

Seizure Log

Possible Triggers

High temperature		Illness or infection	
Missed or late medication		Temperature change	
Overtired		Missed or Poor Sleep	
Mood Change		Fast Breathing	
Missed Meal		Specific Food	
During Sleep		Upon Waking	
Time of day		Screen Use	
Low blood sugar		Low blood sodium	
OTC medications or supplements (please list)		Exercise (What did your child do?)	
Strong emotions - anxiety, stress, excitement, anger. Please describe:		Sensory - sounds, bright colours, flashing lights, patterns. Please describe:	
Other:		Other:	
Other:		Other:	

What happened after? (Recovery Period)

Muscle weakness		Blurred or double vision	
Speech changes		Confusion	
Tired or sleepy		Remembers the event	
Shaking / tremors		Feeling light-headed	
Problems communicating		Unsteady walking	
Loss of coordination (clumsy)		Change in appetite	
Digestive problems		Nausea / Vomiting	
Change in mood: depression, agitation, anger, irritability, excitability		Numbness (name part of body)	
Change in behaviour (detail in notes)		Headache	
Other:		Other:	
Other:		Other:	

Seizure Log

Date: Time: Duration:

Location:

Seizure Type:

If this was a cluster how many seizures?

Child's Mood:

What happened during the seizure?

What was happening around the time the seizure occurred?

Was there an Aura or warning? Yes ☐ No ☐ Describe:

Rescue medication if given:

VNS applied? Yes ☐ No ☐ Detail:

How long did it take your child to recover?

Notes:

Seizure Log

Possible Triggers			
High temperature		Illness or infection	
Missed or late medication		Temperature change	
Overtired		Missed or Poor Sleep	
Mood Change		Fast Breathing	
Missed Meal		Specific Food	
During Sleep		Upon Waking	
Time of day		Screen Use	
Low blood sugar		Low blood sodium	
OTC medications or supplements (please list)		Exercise (What did your child do?)	
Strong emotions - anxiety, stress, excitement, anger. Please describe:		Sensory - sounds, bright colours, flashing lights, patterns. Please describe:	
Other:		Other:	
Other:		Other:	

What happened after? (Recovery Period)			
Muscle weakness		Blurred or double vision	
Speech changes		Confusion	
Tired or sleepy		Remembers the event	
Shaking / tremors		Feeling light-headed	
Problems communicating		Unsteady walking	
Loss of coordination (clumsy)		Change in appetite	
Digestive problems		Nausea / Vomiting	
Change in mood: depression, agitation, anger, irritability, excitability		Numbness (name part of body)	
Change in behaviour (detail in notes)		Headache	
Other:		Other:	
Other:		Other:	

Seizure Log

Date: _____ Time: _____ Duration: _____

Location: _____

Seizure Type: _____

If this was a cluster how many seizures? _____

Child's Mood: _____

What happened during the seizure?
_____
_____
_____
_____

What was happening around the time the seizure occurred?
_____
_____
_____

Was there an Aura or warning? Yes ☐ No ☐ Describe: _____
_____

Rescue medication if given: _____

VNS applied? Yes ☐ No ☐ Detail: _____

How long did it take your child to recover? _____

Notes:
_____
_____
_____
_____

Seizure Log

Possible Triggers			
High temperature		Illness or infection	
Missed or late medication		Temperature change	
Overtired		Missed or Poor Sleep	
Mood Change		Fast Breathing	
Missed Meal		Specific Food	
During Sleep		Upon Waking	
Time of day		Screen Use	
Low blood sugar		Low blood sodium	
OTC medications or supplements (please list)		Exercise (What did your child do?)	
Strong emotions - anxiety, stress, excitement, anger. Please describe:		Sensory - sounds, bright colours, flashing lights, patterns. Please describe:	
Other:		Other:	
Other:		Other:	

What happened after? (Recovery Period)			
Muscle weakness		Blurred or double vision	
Speech changes		Confusion	
Tired or sleepy		Remembers the event	
Shaking / tremors		Feeling light-headed	
Problems communicating		Unsteady walking	
Loss of coordination (clumsy)		Change in appetite	
Digestive problems		Nausea / Vomiting	
Change in mood: depression, agitation, anger, irritability, excitability		Numbness (name part of body)	
Change in behaviour (detail in notes)		Headache	
Other:		Other:	
Other:		Other:	

Seizure Log

Date: Time: Duration:

Location:

Seizure Type:

If this was a cluster how many seizures?

Child's Mood:

What happened during the seizure?

What was happening around the time the seizure occurred?

Was there an Aura or warning? Yes ☐ No ☐ Describe:

Rescue medication if given:

VNS applied? Yes ☐ No ☐ Detail:

How long did it take your child to recover?

Notes:

Seizure Log

Possible Triggers			
High temperature		Illness or infection	
Missed or late medication		Temperature change	
Overtired		Missed or Poor Sleep	
Mood Change		Fast Breathing	
Missed Meal		Specific Food	
During Sleep		Upon Waking	
Time of day		Screen Use	
Low blood sugar		Low blood sodium	
OTC medications or supplements (please list)		Exercise (What did your child do?)	
Strong emotions - anxiety, stress, excitement, anger. Please describe:		Sensory - sounds, bright colours, flashing lights, patterns. Please describe:	
Other:		Other:	
Other:		Other:	

What happened after? (Recovery Period)			
Muscle weakness		Blurred or double vision	
Speech changes		Confusion	
Tired or sleepy		Remembers the event	
Shaking / tremors		Feeling light-headed	
Problems communicating		Unsteady walking	
Loss of coordination (clumsy)		Change in appetite	
Digestive problems		Nausea / Vomiting	
Change in mood: depression, agitation, anger, irritability, excitability		Numbness (name part of body)	
Change in behaviour (detail in notes)		Headache	
Other:		Other:	
Other:		Other:	

Seizure Log

Date: Time: Duration:

Location:

Seizure Type:

If this was a cluster how many seizures?

Child's Mood:

What happened during the seizure?

What was happening around the time the seizure occurred?

Was there an Aura or warning?   Yes ☐   No ☐   Describe:

Rescue medication if given:

VNS applied? Yes ☐   No ☐   Detail:

How long did it take your child to recover?

Notes:

Seizure Log

Possible Triggers			
High temperature		Illness or infection	
Missed or late medication		Temperature change	
Overtired		Missed or Poor Sleep	
Mood Change		Fast Breathing	
Missed Meal		Specific Food	
During Sleep		Upon Waking	
Time of day		Screen Use	
Low blood sugar		Low blood sodium	
OTC medications or supplements (please list)		Exercise (What did your child do?)	
Strong emotions - anxiety, stress, excitement, anger. Please describe:		Sensory - sounds, bright colours, flashing lights, patterns. Please describe:	
Other:		Other:	
Other:		Other:	

What happened after? (Recovery Period)			
Muscle weakness		Blurred or double vision	
Speech changes		Confusion	
Tired or sleepy		Remembers the event	
Shaking / tremors		Feeling light-headed	
Problems communicating		Unsteady walking	
Loss of coordination (clumsy)		Change in appetite	
Digestive problems		Nausea / Vomiting	
Change in mood: depression, agitation, anger, irritability, excitability		Numbness (name part of body)	
Change in behaviour (detail in notes)		Headache	
Other:		Other:	
Other:		Other:	

Seizure Log

Date: Time: Duration:

Location:

Seizure Type:

If this was a cluster how many seizures?

Child's Mood:

What happened during the seizure?

What was happening around the time the seizure occurred?

Was there an Aura or warning? Yes ☐ No ☐ Describe:

Rescue medication if given:

VNS applied? Yes ☐ No ☐ Detail:

How long did it take your child to recover?

Notes:

Seizure Log

Possible Triggers			
High temperature		Illness or infection	
Missed or late medication		Temperature change	
Overtired		Missed or Poor Sleep	
Mood Change		Fast Breathing	
Missed Meal		Specific Food	
During Sleep		Upon Waking	
Time of day		Screen Use	
Low blood sugar		Low blood sodium	
OTC medications or supplements (please list)		Exercise (What did your child do?)	
Strong emotions - anxiety, stress, excitement, anger. Please describe:		Sensory - sounds, bright colours, flashing lights, patterns. Please describe:	
Other:		Other:	
Other:		Other:	

What happened after? (Recovery Period)			
Muscle weakness		Blurred or double vision	
Speech changes		Confusion	
Tired or sleepy		Remembers the event	
Shaking / tremors		Feeling light-headed	
Problems communicating		Unsteady walking	
Loss of coordination (clumsy)		Change in appetite	
Digestive problems		Nausea / Vomiting	
Change in mood: depression, agitation, anger, irritability, excitability		Numbness (name part of body)	
Change in behaviour (detail in notes)		Headache	
Other:		Other:	
Other:		Other:	

Seizure Log

Date: Time: Duration:

Location:

Seizure Type:

If this was a cluster how many seizures?

Child's Mood:

What happened during the seizure?

What was happening around the time the seizure occurred?

Was there an Aura or warning? Yes ☐ No ☐ Describe:

Rescue medication if given:

VNS applied? Yes ☐ No ☐ Detail:

How long did it take your child to recover?

Notes:

Seizure Log

Possible Triggers			
High temperature		Illness or infection	
Missed or late medication		Temperature change	
Overtired		Missed or Poor Sleep	
Mood Change		Fast Breathing	
Missed Meal		Specific Food	
During Sleep		Upon Waking	
Time of day		Screen Use	
Low blood sugar		Low blood sodium	
OTC medications or supplements (please list)		Exercise (What did your child do?)	
Strong emotions - anxiety, stress, excitement, anger. Please describe:		Sensory - sounds, bright colours, flashing lights, patterns. Please describe:	
Other:		Other:	
Other:		Other:	

What happened after? (Recovery Period)			
Muscle weakness		Blurred or double vision	
Speech changes		Confusion	
Tired or sleepy		Remembers the event	
Shaking / tremors		Feeling light-headed	
Problems communicating		Unsteady walking	
Loss of coordination (clumsy)		Change in appetite	
Digestive problems		Nausea / Vomiting	
Change in mood: depression, agitation, anger, irritability, excitability		Numbness (name part of body)	
Change in behaviour (detail in notes)		Headache	
Other:		Other:	
Other:		Other:	

Seizure Log

Date: Time: Duration:

Location:

Seizure Type:

If this was a cluster how many seizures?

Child's Mood:

What happened during the seizure?

What was happening around the time the seizure occurred?

Was there an Aura or warning? Yes ☐ No ☐ Describe:

Rescue medication if given:

VNS applied? Yes ☐ No ☐ Detail:

How long did it take your child to recover?

Notes:

Seizure Log

Possible Triggers			
High temperature		Illness or infection	
Missed or late medication		Temperature change	
Overtired		Missed or Poor Sleep	
Mood Change		Fast Breathing	
Missed Meal		Specific Food	
During Sleep		Upon Waking	
Time of day		Screen Use	
Low blood sugar		Low blood sodium	
OTC medications or supplements (please list)		Exercise (What did your child do?)	
Strong emotions - anxiety, stress, excitement, anger. Please describe:		Sensory - sounds, bright colours, flashing lights, patterns. Please describe:	
Other:		Other:	
Other:		Other:	

What happened after? (Recovery Period)			
Muscle weakness		Blurred or double vision	
Speech changes		Confusion	
Tired or sleepy		Remembers the event	
Shaking / tremors		Feeling light-headed	
Problems communicating		Unsteady walking	
Loss of coordination (clumsy)		Change in appetite	
Digestive problems		Nausea / Vomiting	
Change in mood: depression, agitation, anger, irritability, excitability		Numbness (name part of body)	
Change in behaviour (detail in notes)		Headache	
Other:		Other:	
Other:		Other:	

Seizure Log

Date: Time: Duration:

Location:

Seizure Type:

If this was a cluster how many seizures?

Child's Mood:

What happened during the seizure?

What was happening around the time the seizure occurred?

Was there an Aura or warning? Yes ☐ No ☐ Describe:

Rescue medication if given:

VNS applied? Yes ☐ No ☐ Detail:

How long did it take your child to recover?

Notes:

Seizure Log

Possible Triggers			
High temperature		Illness or infection	
Missed or late medication		Temperature change	
Overtired		Missed or Poor Sleep	
Mood Change		Fast Breathing	
Missed Meal		Specific Food	
During Sleep		Upon Waking	
Time of day		Screen Use	
Low blood sugar		Low blood sodium	
OTC medications or supplements (please list)		Exercise (What did your child do?)	
Strong emotions - anxiety, stress, excitement, anger. Please describe:		Sensory - sounds, bright colours, flashing lights, patterns. Please describe:	
Other:		Other:	
Other:		Other:	

What happened after? (Recovery Period)			
Muscle weakness		Blurred or double vision	
Speech changes		Confusion	
Tired or sleepy		Remembers the event	
Shaking / tremors		Feeling light-headed	
Problems communicating		Unsteady walking	
Loss of coordination (clumsy)		Change in appetite	
Digestive problems		Nausea / Vomiting	
Change in mood: depression, agitation, anger, irritability, excitability		Numbness (name part of body)	
Change in behaviour (detail in notes)		Headache	
Other:		Other:	
Other:		Other:	

Seizure Log

Date: Time: Duration:

Location:

Seizure Type:

If this was a cluster how many seizures?

Child's Mood:

What happened during the seizure?

What was happening around the time the seizure occurred?

Was there an Aura or warning? Yes ☐ No ☐ Describe:

Rescue medication if given:

VNS applied? Yes ☐ No ☐ Detail:

How long did it take your child to recover?

Notes:

Seizure Log

Possible Triggers

High temperature		Illness or infection	
Missed or late medication		Temperature change	
Overtired		Missed or Poor Sleep	
Mood Change		Fast Breathing	
Missed Meal		Specific Food	
During Sleep		Upon Waking	
Time of day		Screen Use	
Low blood sugar		Low blood sodium	
OTC medications or supplements (please list)		Exercise (What did your child do?)	
Strong emotions - anxiety, stress, excitement, anger. Please describe:		Sensory - sounds, bright colours, flashing lights, patterns. Please describe:	
Other:		Other:	
Other:		Other:	

What happened after? (Recovery Period)

Muscle weakness		Blurred or double vision	
Speech changes		Confusion	
Tired or sleepy		Remembers the event	
Shaking / tremors		Feeling light-headed	
Problems communicating		Unsteady walking	
Loss of coordination (clumsy)		Change in appetite	
Digestive problems		Nausea / Vomiting	
Change in mood: depression, agitation, anger, irritability, excitability		Numbness (name part of body)	
Change in behaviour (detail in notes)		Headache	
Other:		Other:	
Other:		Other:	

Seizure Log

Date: Time: Duration:

Location:

Seizure Type:

If this was a cluster how many seizures?

Child's Mood:

What happened during the seizure?

What was happening around the time the seizure occurred?

Was there an Aura or warning? Yes ☐ No ☐ Describe:

Rescue medication if given:

VNS applied? Yes ☐ No ☐ Detail:

How long did it take your child to recover?

Notes:

Seizure Log

Possible Triggers			
High temperature		Illness or infection	
Missed or late medication		Temperature change	
Overtired		Missed or Poor Sleep	
Mood Change		Fast Breathing	
Missed Meal		Specific Food	
During Sleep		Upon Waking	
Time of day		Screen Use	
Low blood sugar		Low blood sodium	
OTC medications or supplements (please list)		Exercise (What did your child do?)	
Strong emotions - anxiety, stress, excitement, anger. Please describe:		Sensory - sounds, bright colours, flashing lights, patterns. Please describe:	
Other:		Other:	
Other:		Other:	

What happened after? (Recovery Period)			
Muscle weakness		Blurred or double vision	
Speech changes		Confusion	
Tired or sleepy		Remembers the event	
Shaking / tremors		Feeling light-headed	
Problems communicating		Unsteady walking	
Loss of coordination (clumsy)		Change in appetite	
Digestive problems		Nausea / Vomiting	
Change in mood: depression, agitation, anger, irritability, excitability		Numbness (name part of body)	
Change in behaviour (detail in notes)		Headache	
Other:		Other:	
Other:		Other:	

Seizure Log

Date: Time: Duration:

Location:

Seizure Type:

If this was a cluster how many seizures?

Child's Mood:

What happened during the seizure?

What was happening around the time the seizure occurred?

Was there an Aura or warning?   Yes ☐   No ☐   Describe:

Rescue medication if given:

VNS applied? Yes ☐   No ☐   Detail:

How long did it take your child to recover?

Notes:

Seizure Log

Possible Triggers			
High temperature		Illness or infection	
Missed or late medication		Temperature change	
Overtired		Missed or Poor Sleep	
Mood Change		Fast Breathing	
Missed Meal		Specific Food	
During Sleep		Upon Waking	
Time of day		Screen Use	
Low blood sugar		Low blood sodium	
OTC medications or supplements (please list)		Exercise (What did your child do?)	
Strong emotions - anxiety, stress, excitement, anger. Please describe:		Sensory - sounds, bright colours, flashing lights, patterns. Please describe:	
Other:		Other:	
Other:		Other:	

What happened after? (Recovery Period)			
Muscle weakness		Blurred or double vision	
Speech changes		Confusion	
Tired or sleepy		Remembers the event	
Shaking / tremors		Feeling light-headed	
Problems communicating		Unsteady walking	
Loss of coordination (clumsy)		Change in appetite	
Digestive problems		Nausea / Vomiting	
Change in mood: depression, agitation, anger, irritability, excitability		Numbness (name part of body)	
Change in behaviour (detail in notes)		Headache	
Other:		Other:	
Other:		Other:	

Seizure Log

Date: _____ Time: _____ Duration: _____

Location: _____

Seizure Type: _____

If this was a cluster how many seizures? _____

Child's Mood: _____

What happened during the seizure?
_____
_____
_____

What was happening around the time the seizure occurred?
_____
_____
_____

Was there an Aura or warning? Yes ☐ No ☐ Describe: _____
_____

Rescue medication if given: _____

VNS applied? Yes ☐ No ☐ Detail: _____

How long did it take your child to recover? _____

Notes:
_____
_____
_____

Seizure Log

Possible Triggers			
High temperature		Illness or infection	
Missed or late medication		Temperature change	
Overtired		Missed or Poor Sleep	
Mood Change		Fast Breathing	
Missed Meal		Specific Food	
During Sleep		Upon Waking	
Time of day		Screen Use	
Low blood sugar		Low blood sodium	
OTC medications or supplements (please list)		Exercise (What did your child do?)	
Strong emotions - anxiety, stress, excitement, anger. Please describe:		Sensory - sounds, bright colours, flashing lights, patterns. Please describe:	
Other:		Other:	
Other:		Other:	

What happened after? (Recovery Period)			
Muscle weakness		Blurred or double vision	
Speech changes		Confusion	
Tired or sleepy		Remembers the event	
Shaking / tremors		Feeling light-headed	
Problems communicating		Unsteady walking	
Loss of coordination (clumsy)		Change in appetite	
Digestive problems		Nausea / Vomiting	
Change in mood: depression, agitation, anger, irritability, excitability		Numbness (name part of body)	
Change in behaviour (detail in notes)		Headache	
Other:		Other:	
Other:		Other:	

Seizure Log

Date: _____   Time: _____   Duration: _____

Location: _____

Seizure Type: _____

If this was a cluster how many seizures? _____

Child's Mood: _____

What happened during the seizure? _____

What was happening around the time the seizure occurred? _____

Was there an Aura or warning? Yes ☐   No ☐   Describe: _____

Rescue medication if given: _____

VNS applied? Yes ☐   No ☐   Detail: _____

How long did it take your child to recover? _____

Notes: _____

Seizure Log

Possible Triggers			
High temperature		Illness or infection	
Missed or late medication		Temperature change	
Overtired		Missed or Poor Sleep	
Mood Change		Fast Breathing	
Missed Meal		Specific Food	
During Sleep		Upon Waking	
Time of day		Screen Use	
Low blood sugar		Low blood sodium	
OTC medications or supplements (please list)		Exercise (What did your child do?)	
Strong emotions - anxiety, stress, excitement, anger. Please describe:		Sensory - sounds, bright colours, flashing lights, patterns. Please describe:	
Other:		Other:	
Other:		Other:	

What happened after? (Recovery Period)			
Muscle weakness		Blurred or double vision	
Speech changes		Confusion	
Tired or sleepy		Remembers the event	
Shaking / tremors		Feeling light-headed	
Problems communicating		Unsteady walking	
Loss of coordination (clumsy)		Change in appetite	
Digestive problems		Nausea / Vomiting	
Change in mood: depression, agitation, anger, irritability, excitability		Numbness (name part of body)	
Change in behaviour (detail in notes)		Headache	
Other:		Other:	
Other:		Other:	

Seizure Log

Date: _____ Time: _____ Duration: _____

Location: _____

Seizure Type: _____

If this was a cluster how many seizures? _____

Child's Mood: _____

What happened during the seizure? _____
_____
_____
_____
_____

What was happening around the time the seizure occurred? _____
_____
_____
_____

Was there an Aura or warning? Yes ☐ No ☐ Describe: _____
_____

Rescue medication if given: _____

VNS applied? Yes ☐ No ☐ Detail: _____

How long did it take your child to recover? _____

Notes: _____
_____
_____
_____
_____

Seizure Log

Possible Triggers			
High temperature		Illness or infection	
Missed or late medication		Temperature change	
Overtired		Missed or Poor Sleep	
Mood Change		Fast Breathing	
Missed Meal		Specific Food	
During Sleep		Upon Waking	
Time of day		Screen Use	
Low blood sugar		Low blood sodium	
OTC medications or supplements (please list)		Exercise (What did your child do?)	
Strong emotions - anxiety, stress, excitement, anger. Please describe:		Sensory - sounds, bright colours, flashing lights, patterns. Please describe:	
Other:		Other:	
Other:		Other:	

What happened after? (Recovery Period)			
Muscle weakness		Blurred or double vision	
Speech changes		Confusion	
Tired or sleepy		Remembers the event	
Shaking / tremors		Feeling light-headed	
Problems communicating		Unsteady walking	
Loss of coordination (clumsy)		Change in appetite	
Digestive problems		Nausea / Vomiting	
Change in mood: depression, agitation, anger, irritability, excitability		Numbness (name part of body)	
Change in behaviour (detail in notes)		Headache	
Other:		Other:	
Other:		Other:	

Seizure Log

Date:　　　　　　　　　　　Time:　　　　　　　　　　Duration:

Location:

Seizure Type:

If this was a cluster how many seizures?

Child's Mood:

What happened during the seizure?

What was happening around the time the seizure occurred?

Was there an Aura or warning? Yes ☐ No ☐ Describe:

Rescue medication if given:

VNS applied? Yes ☐ No ☐ Detail:

How long did it take your child to recover?

Notes:

Seizure Log

Possible Triggers			
High temperature		Illness or infection	
Missed or late medication		Temperature change	
Overtired		Missed or Poor Sleep	
Mood Change		Fast Breathing	
Missed Meal		Specific Food	
During Sleep		Upon Waking	
Time of day		Screen Use	
Low blood sugar		Low blood sodium	
OTC medications or supplements (please list)		Exercise (What did your child do?)	
Strong emotions - anxiety, stress, excitement, anger. Please describe:		Sensory - sounds, bright colours, flashing lights, patterns. Please describe:	
Other:		Other:	
Other:		Other:	

What happened after? (Recovery Period)			
Muscle weakness		Blurred or double vision	
Speech changes		Confusion	
Tired or sleepy		Remembers the event	
Shaking / tremors		Feeling light-headed	
Problems communicating		Unsteady walking	
Loss of coordination (clumsy)		Change in appetite	
Digestive problems		Nausea / Vomiting	
Change in mood: depression, agitation, anger, irritability, excitability		Numbness (name part of body)	
Change in behaviour (detail in notes)		Headache	
Other:		Other:	
Other:		Other:	

Seizure Log

Date: Time: Duration:

Location:

Seizure Type:

If this was a cluster how many seizures?

Child's Mood:

What happened during the seizure?

What was happening around the time the seizure occurred?

Was there an Aura or warning? Yes ☐ No ☐ Describe:

Rescue medication if given:

VNS applied? Yes ☐ No ☐ Detail:

How long did it take your child to recover?

Notes:

Seizure Log

Possible Triggers			
High temperature		Illness or infection	
Missed or late medication		Temperature change	
Overtired		Missed or Poor Sleep	
Mood Change		Fast Breathing	
Missed Meal		Specific Food	
During Sleep		Upon Waking	
Time of day		Screen Use	
Low blood sugar		Low blood sodium	
OTC medications or supplements (please list)		Exercise (What did your child do?)	
Strong emotions - anxiety, stress, excitement, anger. Please describe:		Sensory - sounds, bright colours, flashing lights, patterns. Please describe:	
Other:		Other:	
Other:		Other:	

What happened after? (Recovery Period)			
Muscle weakness		Blurred or double vision	
Speech changes		Confusion	
Tired or sleepy		Remembers the event	
Shaking / tremors		Feeling light-headed	
Problems communicating		Unsteady walking	
Loss of coordination (clumsy)		Change in appetite	
Digestive problems		Nausea / Vomiting	
Change in mood: depression, agitation, anger, irritability, excitability		Numbness (name part of body)	
Change in behaviour (detail in notes)		Headache	
Other:		Other:	
Other:		Other:	

Seizure Log

Date: _____ Time: _____ Duration: _____

Location: _____

Seizure Type: _____

If this was a cluster how many seizures? _____

Child's Mood: _____

What happened during the seizure? _____

_____

_____

_____

What was happening around the time the seizure occurred? _____

_____

_____

Was there an Aura or warning? Yes ☐ No ☐ Describe: _____

_____

Rescue medication if given: _____

VNS applied? Yes ☐ No ☐ Detail: _____

How long did it take your child to recover? _____

Notes: _____

_____

_____

_____

Seizure Log

Possible Triggers			
High temperature		Illness or infection	
Missed or late medication		Temperature change	
Overtired		Missed or Poor Sleep	
Mood Change		Fast Breathing	
Missed Meal		Specific Food	
During Sleep		Upon Waking	
Time of day		Screen Use	
Low blood sugar		Low blood sodium	
OTC medications or supplements (please list)		Exercise (What did your child do?)	
Strong emotions - anxiety, stress, excitement, anger. Please describe:		Sensory - sounds, bright colours, flashing lights, patterns. Please describe:	
Other:		Other:	
Other:		Other:	

What happened after? (Recovery Period)			
Muscle weakness		Blurred or double vision	
Speech changes		Confusion	
Tired or sleepy		Remembers the event	
Shaking / tremors		Feeling light-headed	
Problems communicating		Unsteady walking	
Loss of coordination (clumsy)		Change in appetite	
Digestive problems		Nausea / Vomiting	
Change in mood: depression, agitation, anger, irritability, excitability		Numbness (name part of body)	
Change in behaviour (detail in notes)		Headache	
Other:		Other:	
Other:		Other:	

Seizure Log

Date: Time: Duration:

Location:

Seizure Type:

If this was a cluster how many seizures?

Child's Mood:

What happened during the seizure?

What was happening around the time the seizure occurred?

Was there an Aura or warning? Yes ☐ No ☐ Describe:

Rescue medication if given:

VNS applied? Yes ☐ No ☐ Detail:

How long did it take your child to recover?

Notes:

Seizure Log

Possible Triggers			
High temperature		Illness or infection	
Missed or late medication		Temperature change	
Overtired		Missed or Poor Sleep	
Mood Change		Fast Breathing	
Missed Meal		Specific Food	
During Sleep		Upon Waking	
Time of day		Screen Use	
Low blood sugar		Low blood sodium	
OTC medications or supplements (please list)		Exercise (What did your child do?)	
Strong emotions - anxiety, stress, excitement, anger. Please describe:		Sensory - sounds, bright colours, flashing lights, patterns. Please describe:	
Other:		Other:	
Other:		Other:	

What happened after? (Recovery Period)			
Muscle weakness		Blurred or double vision	
Speech changes		Confusion	
Tired or sleepy		Remembers the event	
Shaking / tremors		Feeling light-headed	
Problems communicating		Unsteady walking	
Loss of coordination (clumsy)		Change in appetite	
Digestive problems		Nausea / Vomiting	
Change in mood: depression, agitation, anger, irritability, excitability		Numbness (name part of body)	
Change in behaviour (detail in notes)		Headache	
Other:		Other:	
Other:		Other:	

Seizure Log

Date: _____ Time: _____ Duration: _____

Location: _____

Seizure Type: _____

If this was a cluster how many seizures? _____

Child's Mood: _____

What happened during the seizure? _____

_____

_____

_____

What was happening around the time the seizure occurred? _____

_____

_____

Was there an Aura or warning? Yes ☐   No ☐   Describe: _____

_____

Rescue medication if given: _____

VNS applied? Yes ☐   No ☐   Detail: _____

_____

How long did it take your child to recover? _____

Notes: _____

_____

_____

_____

Seizure Log

Possible Triggers			
High temperature		Illness or infection	
Missed or late medication		Temperature change	
Overtired		Missed or Poor Sleep	
Mood Change		Fast Breathing	
Missed Meal		Specific Food	
During Sleep		Upon Waking	
Time of day		Screen Use	
Low blood sugar		Low blood sodium	
OTC medications or supplements (please list)		Exercise (What did your child do?)	
Strong emotions - anxiety, stress, excitement, anger. Please describe:		Sensory - sounds, bright colours, flashing lights, patterns. Please describe:	
Other:		Other:	
Other:		Other:	

What happened after? (Recovery Period)			
Muscle weakness		Blurred or double vision	
Speech changes		Confusion	
Tired or sleepy		Remembers the event	
Shaking / tremors		Feeling light-headed	
Problems communicating		Unsteady walking	
Loss of coordination (clumsy)		Change in appetite	
Digestive problems		Nausea / Vomiting	
Change in mood: depression, agitation, anger, irritability, excitability		Numbness (name part of body)	
Change in behaviour (detail in notes)		Headache	
Other:		Other:	
Other:		Other:	

Seizure Log

Date: Time: Duration:

Location:

Seizure Type:

If this was a cluster how many seizures?

Child's Mood:

What happened during the seizure?

What was happening around the time the seizure occurred?

Was there an Aura or warning? Yes ☐ No ☐ Describe:

Rescue medication if given:

VNS applied? Yes ☐ No ☐ Detail:

How long did it take your child to recover?

Notes:

Seizure Log

Possible Triggers			
High temperature		Illness or infection	
Missed or late medication		Temperature change	
Overtired		Missed or Poor Sleep	
Mood Change		Fast Breathing	
Missed Meal		Specific Food	
During Sleep		Upon Waking	
Time of day		Screen Use	
Low blood sugar		Low blood sodium	
OTC medications or supplements (please list)		Exercise (What did your child do?)	
Strong emotions - anxiety, stress, excitement, anger. Please describe:		Sensory - sounds, bright colours, flashing lights, patterns. Please describe:	
Other:		Other:	
Other:		Other:	

What happened after? (Recovery Period)			
Muscle weakness		Blurred or double vision	
Speech changes		Confusion	
Tired or sleepy		Remembers the event	
Shaking / tremors		Feeling light-headed	
Problems communicating		Unsteady walking	
Loss of coordination (clumsy)		Change in appetite	
Digestive problems		Nausea / Vomiting	
Change in mood: depression, agitation, anger, irritability, excitability		Numbness (name part of body)	
Change in behaviour (detail in notes)		Headache	
Other:		Other:	
Other:		Other:	

Seizure Log

Date: _____ Time: _____ Duration: _____

Location: _____

Seizure Type: _____

If this was a cluster how many seizures? _____

Child's Mood: _____

What happened during the seizure? _____

What was happening around the time the seizure occurred? _____

Was there an Aura or warning? Yes ☐ No ☐ Describe: _____

Rescue medication if given: _____

VNS applied? Yes ☐ No ☐ Detail: _____

How long did it take your child to recover? _____

Notes:

Seizure Log

Possible Triggers			
High temperature		Illness or infection	
Missed or late medication		Temperature change	
Overtired		Missed or Poor Sleep	
Mood Change		Fast Breathing	
Missed Meal		Specific Food	
During Sleep		Upon Waking	
Time of day		Screen Use	
Low blood sugar		Low blood sodium	
OTC medications or supplements (please list)		Exercise (What did your child do?)	
Strong emotions - anxiety, stress, excitement, anger. Please describe:		Sensory - sounds, bright colours, flashing lights, patterns. Please describe:	
Other:		Other:	
Other:		Other:	

What happened after? (Recovery Period)			
Muscle weakness		Blurred or double vision	
Speech changes		Confusion	
Tired or sleepy		Remembers the event	
Shaking / tremors		Feeling light-headed	
Problems communicating		Unsteady walking	
Loss of coordination (clumsy)		Change in appetite	
Digestive problems		Nausea / Vomiting	
Change in mood: depression, agitation, anger, irritability, excitability		Numbness (name part of body)	
Change in behaviour (detail in notes)		Headache	
Other:		Other:	
Other:		Other:	

Seizure Log

Date: _____ Time: _____ Duration: _____

Location: _____

Seizure Type: _____

If this was a cluster how many seizures? _____

Child's Mood: _____

What happened during the seizure? _____

_____

_____

_____

What was happening around the time the seizure occurred? _____

_____

_____

Was there an Aura or warning? Yes ☐ No ☐ Describe: _____

_____

Rescue medication if given: _____

VNS applied? Yes ☐ No ☐ Detail: _____

How long did it take your child to recover? _____

Notes: _____

_____

_____

_____

Seizure Log

Possible Triggers			
High temperature		Illness or infection	
Missed or late medication		Temperature change	
Overtired		Missed or Poor Sleep	
Mood Change		Fast Breathing	
Missed Meal		Specific Food	
During Sleep		Upon Waking	
Time of day		Screen Use	
Low blood sugar		Low blood sodium	
OTC medications or supplements (please list)		Exercise (What did your child do?)	
Strong emotions - anxiety, stress, excitement, anger. Please describe:		Sensory - sounds, bright colours, flashing lights, patterns. Please describe:	
Other:		Other:	
Other:		Other:	

What happened after? (Recovery Period)			
Muscle weakness		Blurred or double vision	
Speech changes		Confusion	
Tired or sleepy		Remembers the event	
Shaking / tremors		Feeling light-headed	
Problems communicating		Unsteady walking	
Loss of coordination (clumsy)		Change in appetite	
Digestive problems		Nausea / Vomiting	
Change in mood: depression, agitation, anger, irritability, excitability		Numbness (name part of body)	
Change in behaviour (detail in notes)		Headache	
Other:		Other:	
Other:		Other:	

Seizure Log

Date: Time: Duration:

Location:

Seizure Type:

If this was a cluster how many seizures?

Child's Mood:

What happened during the seizure?

What was happening around the time the seizure occurred?

Was there an Aura or warning? Yes ☐ No ☐ Describe:

Rescue medication if given:

VNS applied? Yes ☐ No ☐ Detail:

How long did it take your child to recover?

Notes:

Seizure Log

Possible Triggers			
High temperature		Illness or infection	
Missed or late medication		Temperature change	
Overtired		Missed or Poor Sleep	
Mood Change		Fast Breathing	
Missed Meal		Specific Food	
During Sleep		Upon Waking	
Time of day		Screen Use	
Low blood sugar		Low blood sodium	
OTC medications or supplements (please list)		Exercise (What did your child do?)	
Strong emotions - anxiety, stress, excitement, anger. Please describe:		Sensory - sounds, bright colours, flashing lights, patterns. Please describe:	
Other:		Other:	
Other:		Other:	

What happened after? (Recovery Period)			
Muscle weakness		Blurred or double vision	
Speech changes		Confusion	
Tired or sleepy		Remembers the event	
Shaking / tremors		Feeling light-headed	
Problems communicating		Unsteady walking	
Loss of coordination (clumsy)		Change in appetite	
Digestive problems		Nausea / Vomiting	
Change in mood: depression, agitation, anger, irritability, excitability		Numbness (name part of body)	
Change in behaviour (detail in notes)		Headache	
Other:		Other:	
Other:		Other:	

Seizure Log

Date: Time: Duration:

Location:

Seizure Type:

If this was a cluster how many seizures?

Child's Mood:

What happened during the seizure?

What was happening around the time the seizure occurred?

Was there an Aura or warning? Yes ☐ No ☐ Describe:

Rescue medication if given:

VNS applied? Yes ☐ No ☐ Detail:

How long did it take your child to recover?

Notes:

Seizure Log

Possible Triggers			
High temperature		Illness or infection	
Missed or late medication		Temperature change	
Overtired		Missed or Poor Sleep	
Mood Change		Fast Breathing	
Missed Meal		Specific Food	
During Sleep		Upon Waking	
Time of day		Screen Use	
Low blood sugar		Low blood sodium	
OTC medications or supplements (please list)		Exercise (What did your child do?)	
Strong emotions - anxiety, stress, excitement, anger. Please describe:		Sensory - sounds, bright colours, flashing lights, patterns. Please describe:	
Other:		Other:	
Other:		Other:	

What happened after? (Recovery Period)			
Muscle weakness		Blurred or double vision	
Speech changes		Confusion	
Tired or sleepy		Remembers the event	
Shaking / tremors		Feeling light-headed	
Problems communicating		Unsteady walking	
Loss of coordination (clumsy)		Change in appetite	
Digestive problems		Nausea / Vomiting	
Change in mood: depression, agitation, anger, irritability, excitability		Numbness (name part of body)	
Change in behaviour (detail in notes)		Headache	
Other:		Other:	
Other:		Other:	

Seizure Log

Date: _____ Time: _____ Duration: _____

Location: _____

Seizure Type: _____

If this was a cluster how many seizures? _____

Child's Mood: _____

What happened during the seizure? _____

_____

_____

_____

What was happening around the time the seizure occurred? _____

_____

_____

Was there an Aura or warning? Yes ☐ No ☐ Describe: _____

_____

Rescue medication if given: _____

VNS applied? Yes ☐ No ☐ Detail: _____

How long did it take your child to recover? _____

Notes: _____

_____

_____

_____

Seizure Log

Possible Triggers			
High temperature		Illness or infection	
Missed or late medication		Temperature change	
Overtired		Missed or Poor Sleep	
Mood Change		Fast Breathing	
Missed Meal		Specific Food	
During Sleep		Upon Waking	
Time of day		Screen Use	
Low blood sugar		Low blood sodium	
OTC medications or supplements (please list)		Exercise (What did your child do?)	
Strong emotions - anxiety, stress, excitement, anger. Please describe:		Sensory - sounds, bright colours, flashing lights, patterns. Please describe:	
Other:		Other:	
Other:		Other:	

What happened after? (Recovery Period)			
Muscle weakness		Blurred or double vision	
Speech changes		Confusion	
Tired or sleepy		Remembers the event	
Shaking / tremors		Feeling light-headed	
Problems communicating		Unsteady walking	
Loss of coordination (clumsy)		Change in appetite	
Digestive problems		Nausea / Vomiting	
Change in mood: depression, agitation, anger, irritability, excitability		Numbness (name part of body)	
Change in behaviour (detail in notes)		Headache	
Other:		Other:	
Other:		Other:	

Seizure Log

Date: _____ Time: _____ Duration: _____

Location: _____

Seizure Type: _____

If this was a cluster how many seizures? _____

Child's Mood: _____

What happened during the seizure? _____

_____

_____

_____

What was happening around the time the seizure occurred? _____

_____

_____

Was there an Aura or warning? Yes ☐ No ☐ Describe: _____

_____

Rescue medication if given: _____

VNS applied? Yes ☐ No ☐ Detail: _____

How long did it take your child to recover? _____

Notes: _____

_____

_____

_____

Seizure Log

Possible Triggers			
High temperature		Illness or infection	
Missed or late medication		Temperature change	
Overtired		Missed or Poor Sleep	
Mood Change		Fast Breathing	
Missed Meal		Specific Food	
During Sleep		Upon Waking	
Time of day		Screen Use	
Low blood sugar		Low blood sodium	
OTC medications or supplements (please list)		Exercise (What did your child do?)	
Strong emotions - anxiety, stress, excitement, anger. Please describe:		Sensory - sounds, bright colours, flashing lights, patterns. Please describe:	
Other:		Other:	
Other:		Other:	

What happened after? (Recovery Period)			
Muscle weakness		Blurred or double vision	
Speech changes		Confusion	
Tired or sleepy		Remembers the event	
Shaking / tremors		Feeling light-headed	
Problems communicating		Unsteady walking	
Loss of coordination (clumsy)		Change in appetite	
Digestive problems		Nausea / Vomiting	
Change in mood: depression, agitation, anger, irritability, excitability		Numbness (name part of body)	
Change in behaviour (detail in notes)		Headache	
Other:		Other:	
Other:		Other:	

Seizure Log

Date: Time: Duration:

Location:

Seizure Type:

If this was a cluster how many seizures?

Child's Mood:

What happened during the seizure?

What was happening around the time the seizure occurred?

Was there an Aura or warning? Yes ☐ No ☐ Describe:

Rescue medication if given:

VNS applied? Yes ☐ No ☐ Detail:

How long did it take your child to recover?

Notes:

Seizure Log

Possible Triggers				
High temperature		Illness or infection	
Missed or late medication		Temperature change	
Overtired		Missed or Poor Sleep	
Mood Change		Fast Breathing	
Missed Meal		Specific Food	
During Sleep		Upon Waking	
Time of day		Screen Use	
Low blood sugar		Low blood sodium	
OTC medications or supplements (please list)		Exercise (What did your child do?)	
Strong emotions - anxiety, stress, excitement, anger. Please describe:		Sensory - sounds, bright colours, flashing lights, patterns. Please describe:	
Other:		Other:	
Other:		Other:	

What happened after? (Recovery Period)				
Muscle weakness		Blurred or double vision	
Speech changes		Confusion	
Tired or sleepy		Remembers the event	
Shaking / tremors		Feeling light-headed	
Problems communicating		Unsteady walking	
Loss of coordination (clumsy)		Change in appetite	
Digestive problems		Nausea / Vomiting	
Change in mood: depression, agitation, anger, irritability, excitability		Numbness (name part of body)	
Change in behaviour (detail in notes)		Headache	
Other:		Other:	
Other:		Other:	

Seizure Log

Date: _____   Time: _____   Duration: _____

Location: _____

Seizure Type: _____

If this was a cluster how many seizures? _____

Child's Mood: _____

What happened during the seizure? _____

_____

_____

_____

What was happening around the time the seizure occurred? _____

_____

_____

Was there an Aura or warning? Yes ☐   No ☐   Describe: _____

_____

Rescue medication if given: _____

VNS applied? Yes ☐   No ☐   Detail: _____

How long did it take your child to recover? _____

Notes: _____

_____

_____

_____

Seizure Log

Possible Triggers			
High temperature		Illness or infection	
Missed or late medication		Temperature change	
Overtired		Missed or Poor Sleep	
Mood Change		Fast Breathing	
Missed Meal		Specific Food	
During Sleep		Upon Waking	
Time of day		Screen Use	
Low blood sugar		Low blood sodium	
OTC medications or supplements (please list)		Exercise (What did your child do?)	
Strong emotions - anxiety, stress, excitement, anger. Please describe:		Sensory - sounds, bright colours, flashing lights, patterns. Please describe:	
Other:		Other:	
Other:		Other:	

What happened after? (Recovery Period)			
Muscle weakness		Blurred or double vision	
Speech changes		Confusion	
Tired or sleepy		Remembers the event	
Shaking / tremors		Feeling light-headed	
Problems communicating		Unsteady walking	
Loss of coordination (clumsy)		Change in appetite	
Digestive problems		Nausea / Vomiting	
Change in mood: depression, agitation, anger, irritability, excitability		Numbness (name part of body)	
Change in behaviour (detail in notes)		Headache	
Other:		Other:	
Other:		Other:	

Seizure Log

Date: _____ Time: _____ Duration: _____

Location: _____

Seizure Type: _____

If this was a cluster how many seizures? _____

Child's Mood: _____

What happened during the seizure?

_____
_____
_____
_____

What was happening around the time the seizure occurred?

_____
_____
_____
_____

Was there an Aura or warning? Yes ☐ No ☐ Describe: _____

_____

Rescue medication if given: _____

VNS applied? Yes ☐ No ☐ Detail: _____

How long did it take your child to recover? _____

Notes:

_____
_____
_____
_____

Seizure Log

Possible Triggers			
High temperature		Illness or infection	
Missed or late medication		Temperature change	
Overtired		Missed or Poor Sleep	
Mood Change		Fast Breathing	
Missed Meal		Specific Food	
During Sleep		Upon Waking	
Time of day		Screen Use	
Low blood sugar		Low blood sodium	
OTC medications or supplements (please list)		Exercise (What did your child do?)	
Strong emotions - anxiety, stress, excitement, anger. Please describe:		Sensory - sounds, bright colours, flashing lights, patterns. Please describe:	
Other:		Other:	
Other:		Other:	

What happened after? (Recovery Period)			
Muscle weakness		Blurred or double vision	
Speech changes		Confusion	
Tired or sleepy		Remembers the event	
Shaking / tremors		Feeling light-headed	
Problems communicating		Unsteady walking	
Loss of coordination (clumsy)		Change in appetite	
Digestive problems		Nausea / Vomiting	
Change in mood: depression, agitation, anger, irritability, excitability		Numbness (name part of body)	
Change in behaviour (detail in notes)		Headache	
Other:		Other:	
Other:		Other:	

Seizure Log

Date: Time: Duration:

Location:

Seizure Type:

If this was a cluster how many seizures?

Child's Mood:

What happened during the seizure?

What was happening around the time the seizure occurred?

Was there an Aura or warning? Yes ☐ No ☐ Describe:

Rescue medication if given:

VNS applied? Yes ☐ No ☐ Detail:

How long did it take your child to recover?

Notes:

Seizure Log

Possible Triggers			
High temperature		Illness or infection	
Missed or late medication		Temperature change	
Overtired		Missed or Poor Sleep	
Mood Change		Fast Breathing	
Missed Meal		Specific Food	
During Sleep		Upon Waking	
Time of day		Screen Use	
Low blood sugar		Low blood sodium	
OTC medications or supplements (please list)		Exercise (What did your child do?)	
Strong emotions - anxiety, stress, excitement, anger. Please describe:		Sensory - sounds, bright colours, flashing lights, patterns. Please describe:	
Other:		Other:	
Other:		Other:	

What happened after? (Recovery Period)			
Muscle weakness		Blurred or double vision	
Speech changes		Confusion	
Tired or sleepy		Remembers the event	
Shaking / tremors		Feeling light-headed	
Problems communicating		Unsteady walking	
Loss of coordination (clumsy)		Change in appetite	
Digestive problems		Nausea / Vomiting	
Change in mood: depression, agitation, anger, irritability, excitability		Numbness (name part of body)	
Change in behaviour (detail in notes)		Headache	
Other:		Other:	
Other:		Other:	

Seizure Log

Date: _____ Time: _____ Duration: _____

Location: _____

Seizure Type: _____

If this was a cluster how many seizures? _____

Child's Mood: _____

What happened during the seizure? _____

What was happening around the time the seizure occurred? _____

Was there an Aura or warning? Yes ☐ No ☐ Describe: _____

Rescue medication if given: _____

VNS applied? Yes ☐ No ☐ Detail: _____

How long did it take your child to recover? _____

Notes: _____

Seizure Log

Possible Triggers			
High temperature		Illness or infection	
Missed or late medication		Temperature change	
Overtired		Missed or Poor Sleep	
Mood Change		Fast Breathing	
Missed Meal		Specific Food	
During Sleep		Upon Waking	
Time of day		Screen Use	
Low blood sugar		Low blood sodium	
OTC medications or supplements (please list)		Exercise (What did your child do?)	
Strong emotions - anxiety, stress, excitement, anger. Please describe:		Sensory - sounds, bright colours, flashing lights, patterns. Please describe:	
Other:		Other:	
Other:		Other:	

What happened after? (Recovery Period)			
Muscle weakness		Blurred or double vision	
Speech changes		Confusion	
Tired or sleepy		Remembers the event	
Shaking / tremors		Feeling light-headed	
Problems communicating		Unsteady walking	
Loss of coordination (clumsy)		Change in appetite	
Digestive problems		Nausea / Vomiting	
Change in mood: depression, agitation, anger, irritability, excitability		Numbness (name part of body)	
Change in behaviour (detail in notes)		Headache	
Other:		Other:	
Other:		Other:	

Seizure Log

Date: Time: Duration:

Location:

Seizure Type:

If this was a cluster how many seizures?

Child's Mood:

What happened during the seizure?

What was happening around the time the seizure occurred?

Was there an Aura or warning? Yes ☐ No ☐ Describe:

Rescue medication if given:

VNS applied? Yes ☐ No ☐ Detail:

How long did it take your child to recover?

Notes:

Seizure Log

Possible Triggers			
High temperature		Illness or infection	
Missed or late medication		Temperature change	
Overtired		Missed or Poor Sleep	
Mood Change		Fast Breathing	
Missed Meal		Specific Food	
During Sleep		Upon Waking	
Time of day		Screen Use	
Low blood sugar		Low blood sodium	
OTC medications or supplements (please list)		Exercise (What did your child do?)	
Strong emotions - anxiety, stress, excitement, anger. Please describe:		Sensory - sounds, bright colours, flashing lights, patterns. Please describe:	
Other:		Other:	
Other:		Other:	

What happened after? (Recovery Period)			
Muscle weakness		Blurred or double vision	
Speech changes		Confusion	
Tired or sleepy		Remembers the event	
Shaking / tremors		Feeling light-headed	
Problems communicating		Unsteady walking	
Loss of coordination (clumsy)		Change in appetite	
Digestive problems		Nausea / Vomiting	
Change in mood: depression, agitation, anger, irritability, excitability		Numbness (name part of body)	
Change in behaviour (detail in notes)		Headache	
Other:		Other:	
Other:		Other:	

Seizure Log

Date: Time: Duration:

Location:

Seizure Type:

If this was a cluster how many seizures?

Child's Mood:

What happened during the seizure?

What was happening around the time the seizure occurred?

Was there an Aura or warning? Yes ☐ No ☐ Describe:

Rescue medication if given:

VNS applied? Yes ☐ No ☐ Detail:

How long did it take your child to recover?

Notes:

Seizure Log

Possible Triggers			
High temperature		Illness or infection	
Missed or late medication		Temperature change	
Overtired		Missed or Poor Sleep	
Mood Change		Fast Breathing	
Missed Meal		Specific Food	
During Sleep		Upon Waking	
Time of day		Screen Use	
Low blood sugar		Low blood sodium	
OTC medications or supplements (please list)		Exercise (What did your child do?)	
Strong emotions - anxiety, stress, excitement, anger. Please describe:		Sensory - sounds, bright colours, flashing lights, patterns. Please describe:	
Other:		Other:	
Other:		Other:	

What happened after? (Recovery Period)			
Muscle weakness		Blurred or double vision	
Speech changes		Confusion	
Tired or sleepy		Remembers the event	
Shaking / tremors		Feeling light-headed	
Problems communicating		Unsteady walking	
Loss of coordination (clumsy)		Change in appetite	
Digestive problems		Nausea / Vomiting	
Change in mood: depression, agitation, anger, irritability, excitability		Numbness (name part of body)	
Change in behaviour (detail in notes)		Headache	
Other:		Other:	
Other:		Other:	

Seizure Log

Date: _____ Time: _____ Duration: _____

Location: _____

Seizure Type: _____

If this was a cluster how many seizures? _____

Child's Mood: _____

What happened during the seizure? _____

_____

_____

_____

What was happening around the time the seizure occurred? _____

_____

_____

Was there an Aura or warning? Yes ☐ No ☐ Describe: _____

_____

Rescue medication if given: _____

VNS applied? Yes ☐ No ☐ Detail: _____

How long did it take your child to recover? _____

Notes: _____

_____

_____

_____

Seizure Log

Possible Triggers			
High temperature		Illness or infection	
Missed or late medication		Temperature change	
Overtired		Missed or Poor Sleep	
Mood Change		Fast Breathing	
Missed Meal		Specific Food	
During Sleep		Upon Waking	
Time of day		Screen Use	
Low blood sugar		Low blood sodium	
OTC medications or supplements (please list)		Exercise (What did your child do?)	
Strong emotions - anxiety, stress, excitement, anger. Please describe:		Sensory - sounds, bright colours, flashing lights, patterns. Please describe:	
Other:		Other:	
Other:		Other:	

What happened after? (Recovery Period)			
Muscle weakness		Blurred or double vision	
Speech changes		Confusion	
Tired or sleepy		Remembers the event	
Shaking / tremors		Feeling light-headed	
Problems communicating		Unsteady walking	
Loss of coordination (clumsy)		Change in appetite	
Digestive problems		Nausea / Vomiting	
Change in mood: depression, agitation, anger, irritability, excitability		Numbness (name part of body)	
Change in behaviour (detail in notes)		Headache	
Other:		Other:	
Other:		Other:	

Seizure Log

Date: _____   Time: _____   Duration: _____

Location: _____

Seizure Type: _____

If this was a cluster how many seizures? _____

Child's Mood: _____

What happened during the seizure? _____

What was happening around the time the seizure occurred? _____

Was there an Aura or warning?   Yes ☐   No ☐   Describe: _____

Rescue medication if given: _____

VNS applied? Yes ☐   No ☐   Detail: _____

How long did it take your child to recover? _____

Notes: _____

Seizure Log

Possible Triggers			
High temperature		Illness or infection	
Missed or late medication		Temperature change	
Overtired		Missed or Poor Sleep	
Mood Change		Fast Breathing	
Missed Meal		Specific Food	
During Sleep		Upon Waking	
Time of day		Screen Use	
Low blood sugar		Low blood sodium	
OTC medications or supplements (please list)		Exercise (What did your child do?)	
Strong emotions - anxiety, stress, excitement, anger. Please describe:		Sensory - sounds, bright colours, flashing lights, patterns. Please describe:	
Other:		Other:	
Other:		Other:	

What happened after? (Recovery Period)			
Muscle weakness		Blurred or double vision	
Speech changes		Confusion	
Tired or sleepy		Remembers the event	
Shaking / tremors		Feeling light-headed	
Problems communicating		Unsteady walking	
Loss of coordination (clumsy)		Change in appetite	
Digestive problems		Nausea / Vomiting	
Change in mood: depression, agitation, anger, irritability, excitability		Numbness (name part of body)	
Change in behaviour (detail in notes)		Headache	
Other:		Other:	
Other:		Other:	

Seizure Log

Date: Time: Duration:

Location:

Seizure Type:

If this was a cluster how many seizures?

Child's Mood:

What happened during the seizure?

What was happening around the time the seizure occurred?

Was there an Aura or warning? Yes ☐ No ☐ Describe:

Rescue medication if given:

VNS applied? Yes ☐ No ☐ Detail:

How long did it take your child to recover?

Notes:

Seizure Log

Possible Triggers			
High temperature		Illness or infection	
Missed or late medication		Temperature change	
Overtired		Missed or Poor Sleep	
Mood Change		Fast Breathing	
Missed Meal		Specific Food	
During Sleep		Upon Waking	
Time of day		Screen Use	
Low blood sugar		Low blood sodium	
OTC medications or supplements (please list)		Exercise (What did your child do?)	
Strong emotions - anxiety, stress, excitement, anger. Please describe:		Sensory - sounds, bright colours, flashing lights, patterns. Please describe:	
Other:		Other:	
Other:		Other:	

What happened after? (Recovery Period)			
Muscle weakness		Blurred or double vision	
Speech changes		Confusion	
Tired or sleepy		Remembers the event	
Shaking / tremors		Feeling light-headed	
Problems communicating		Unsteady walking	
Loss of coordination (clumsy)		Change in appetite	
Digestive problems		Nausea / Vomiting	
Change in mood: depression, agitation, anger, irritability, excitability		Numbness (name part of body)	
Change in behaviour (detail in notes)		Headache	
Other:		Other:	
Other:		Other:	

Seizure Log

Date: Time: Duration:

Location:

Seizure Type:

If this was a cluster how many seizures?

Child's Mood:

What happened during the seizure?

What was happening around the time the seizure occurred?

Was there an Aura or warning? Yes ☐ No ☐ Describe:

Rescue medication if given:

VNS applied? Yes ☐ No ☐ Detail:

How long did it take your child to recover?

Notes:

Seizure Log

Possible Triggers			
High temperature		Illness or infection	
Missed or late medication		Temperature change	
Overtired		Missed or Poor Sleep	
Mood Change		Fast Breathing	
Missed Meal		Specific Food	
During Sleep		Upon Waking	
Time of day		Screen Use	
Low blood sugar		Low blood sodium	
OTC medications or supplements (please list)		Exercise (What did your child do?)	
Strong emotions - anxiety, stress, excitement, anger. Please describe:		Sensory - sounds, bright colours, flashing lights, patterns. Please describe:	
Other:		Other:	
Other:		Other:	

What happened after? (Recovery Period)			
Muscle weakness		Blurred or double vision	
Speech changes		Confusion	
Tired or sleepy		Remembers the event	
Shaking / tremors		Feeling light-headed	
Problems communicating		Unsteady walking	
Loss of coordination (clumsy)		Change in appetite	
Digestive problems		Nausea / Vomiting	
Change in mood: depression, agitation, anger, irritability, excitability		Numbness (name part of body)	
Change in behaviour (detail in notes)		Headache	
Other:		Other:	
Other:		Other:	

Seizure Log

Date: _____ Time: _____ Duration: _____

Location: _____

Seizure Type: _____

If this was a cluster how many seizures? _____

Child's Mood: _____

What happened during the seizure? _____

_____

_____

_____

What was happening around the time the seizure occurred? _____

_____

_____

Was there an Aura or warning? Yes ☐ No ☐ Describe: _____

_____

Rescue medication if given: _____

VNS applied? Yes ☐ No ☐ Detail: _____

How long did it take your child to recover? _____

Notes: _____

_____

_____

_____

Seizure Log

Possible Triggers			
High temperature		Illness or infection	
Missed or late medication		Temperature change	
Overtired		Missed or Poor Sleep	
Mood Change		Fast Breathing	
Missed Meal		Specific Food	
During Sleep		Upon Waking	
Time of day		Screen Use	
Low blood sugar		Low blood sodium	
OTC medications or supplements (please list)		Exercise (What did your child do?)	
Strong emotions - anxiety, stress, excitement, anger. Please describe:		Sensory - sounds, bright colours, flashing lights, patterns. Please describe:	
Other:		Other:	
Other:		Other:	

What happened after? (Recovery Period)			
Muscle weakness		Blurred or double vision	
Speech changes		Confusion	
Tired or sleepy		Remembers the event	
Shaking / tremors		Feeling light-headed	
Problems communicating		Unsteady walking	
Loss of coordination (clumsy)		Change in appetite	
Digestive problems		Nausea / Vomiting	
Change in mood: depression, agitation, anger, irritability, excitability		Numbness (name part of body)	
Change in behaviour (detail in notes)		Headache	
Other:		Other:	
Other:		Other:	

Seizure Log

Date: _____ Time: _____ Duration: _____

Location: _____

Seizure Type: _____

If this was a cluster how many seizures? _____

Child's Mood: _____

What happened during the seizure?

_____

_____

_____

_____

What was happening around the time the seizure occurred?

_____

_____

_____

Was there an Aura or warning? Yes ☐ No ☐ Describe: _____

_____

Rescue medication if given: _____

VNS applied? Yes ☐ No ☐ Detail: _____

_____

How long did it take your child to recover? _____

Notes:

_____

_____

_____

_____

Seizure Log

Possible Triggers			
High temperature		Illness or infection	
Missed or late medication		Temperature change	
Overtired		Missed or Poor Sleep	
Mood Change		Fast Breathing	
Missed Meal		Specific Food	
During Sleep		Upon Waking	
Time of day		Screen Use	
Low blood sugar		Low blood sodium	
OTC medications or supplements (please list)		Exercise (What did your child do?)	
Strong emotions - anxiety, stress, excitement, anger. Please describe:		Sensory - sounds, bright colours, flashing lights, patterns. Please describe:	
Other:		Other:	
Other:		Other:	

What happened after? (Recovery Period)			
Muscle weakness		Blurred or double vision	
Speech changes		Confusion	
Tired or sleepy		Remembers the event	
Shaking / tremors		Feeling light-headed	
Problems communicating		Unsteady walking	
Loss of coordination (clumsy)		Change in appetite	
Digestive problems		Nausea / Vomiting	
Change in mood: depression, agitation, anger, irritability, excitability		Numbness (name part of body)	
Change in behaviour (detail in notes)		Headache	
Other:		Other:	
Other:		Other:	

Seizure Log

Date: _____ Time: _____ Duration: _____

Location: _____

Seizure Type: _____

If this was a cluster how many seizures? _____

Child's Mood: _____

What happened during the seizure? _____

_____

_____

_____

What was happening around the time the seizure occurred? _____

_____

_____

Was there an Aura or warning? Yes ☐ No ☐ Describe: _____

_____

Rescue medication if given: _____

VNS applied? Yes ☐ No ☐ Detail: _____

How long did it take your child to recover? _____

Notes: _____

_____

_____

_____

Seizure Log

Possible Triggers			
High temperature		Illness or infection	
Missed or late medication		Temperature change	
Overtired		Missed or Poor Sleep	
Mood Change		Fast Breathing	
Missed Meal		Specific Food	
During Sleep		Upon Waking	
Time of day		Screen Use	
Low blood sugar		Low blood sodium	
OTC medications or supplements (please list)		Exercise (What did your child do?)	
Strong emotions - anxiety, stress, excitement, anger. Please describe:		Sensory - sounds, bright colours, flashing lights, patterns. Please describe:	
Other:		Other:	
Other:		Other:	

What happened after? (Recovery Period)			
Muscle weakness		Blurred or double vision	
Speech changes		Confusion	
Tired or sleepy		Remembers the event	
Shaking / tremors		Feeling light-headed	
Problems communicating		Unsteady walking	
Loss of coordination (clumsy)		Change in appetite	
Digestive problems		Nausea / Vomiting	
Change in mood: depression, agitation, anger, irritability, excitability		Numbness (name part of body)	
Change in behaviour (detail in notes)		Headache	
Other:		Other:	
Other:		Other:	

Seizure Log

Date: _____ Time: _____ Duration: _____

Location:

Seizure Type:

If this was a cluster how many seizures?

Child's Mood:

What happened during the seizure?

What was happening around the time the seizure occurred?

Was there an Aura or warning? Yes ☐ No ☐ Describe:

Rescue medication if given:

VNS applied? Yes ☐ No ☐ Detail:

How long did it take your child to recover?

Notes:

Seizure Log

Possible Triggers			
High temperature		Illness or infection	
Missed or late medication		Temperature change	
Overtired		Missed or Poor Sleep	
Mood Change		Fast Breathing	
Missed Meal		Specific Food	
During Sleep		Upon Waking	
Time of day		Screen Use	
Low blood sugar		Low blood sodium	
OTC medications or supplements (please list)		Exercise (What did your child do?)	
Strong emotions - anxiety, stress, excitement, anger. Please describe:		Sensory - sounds, bright colours, flashing lights, patterns. Please describe:	
Other:		Other:	
Other:		Other:	

What happened after? (Recovery Period)			
Muscle weakness		Blurred or double vision	
Speech changes		Confusion	
Tired or sleepy		Remembers the event	
Shaking / tremors		Feeling light-headed	
Problems communicating		Unsteady walking	
Loss of coordination (clumsy)		Change in appetite	
Digestive problems		Nausea / Vomiting	
Change in mood: depression, agitation, anger, irritability, excitability		Numbness (name part of body)	
Change in behaviour (detail in notes)		Headache	
Other:		Other:	
Other:		Other:	

Seizure Log

Date: _____ Time: _____ Duration: _____

Location:

Seizure Type:

If this was a cluster how many seizures?

Child's Mood:

What happened during the seizure?

What was happening around the time the seizure occurred?

Was there an Aura or warning? Yes ☐ No ☐ Describe:

Rescue medication if given:

VNS applied? Yes ☐ No ☐ Detail:

How long did it take your child to recover?

Notes:

Seizure Log

Possible Triggers			
High temperature		Illness or infection	
Missed or late medication		Temperature change	
Overtired		Missed or Poor Sleep	
Mood Change		Fast Breathing	
Missed Meal		Specific Food	
During Sleep		Upon Waking	
Time of day		Screen Use	
Low blood sugar		Low blood sodium	
OTC medications or supplements (please list)		Exercise (What did your child do?)	
Strong emotions - anxiety, stress, excitement, anger. Please describe:		Sensory - sounds, bright colours, flashing lights, patterns. Please describe:	
Other:		Other:	
Other:		Other:	

What happened after? (Recovery Period)			
Muscle weakness		Blurred or double vision	
Speech changes		Confusion	
Tired or sleepy		Remembers the event	
Shaking / tremors		Feeling light-headed	
Problems communicating		Unsteady walking	
Loss of coordination (clumsy)		Change in appetite	
Digestive problems		Nausea / Vomiting	
Change in mood: depression, agitation, anger, irritability, excitability		Numbness (name part of body)	
Change in behaviour (detail in notes)		Headache	
Other:		Other:	
Other:		Other:	

Seizure Log

Date: _____ Time: _____ Duration: _____

Location: _____

Seizure Type: _____

If this was a cluster how many seizures? _____

Child's Mood: _____

What happened during the seizure? _____

_____

_____

_____

What was happening around the time the seizure occurred? _____

_____

_____

Was there an Aura or warning? Yes ☐ No ☐ Describe: _____

_____

Rescue medication if given: _____

VNS applied? Yes ☐ No ☐ Detail: _____

How long did it take your child to recover? _____

Notes: _____

_____

_____

_____

Seizure Log

Possible Triggers			
High temperature		Illness or infection	
Missed or late medication		Temperature change	
Overtired		Missed or Poor Sleep	
Mood Change		Fast Breathing	
Missed Meal		Specific Food	
During Sleep		Upon Waking	
Time of day		Screen Use	
Low blood sugar		Low blood sodium	
OTC medications or supplements (please list)		Exercise (What did your child do?)	
Strong emotions - anxiety, stress, excitement, anger. Please describe:		Sensory - sounds, bright colours, flashing lights, patterns. Please describe:	
Other:		Other:	
Other:		Other:	

What happened after? (Recovery Period)			
Muscle weakness		Blurred or double vision	
Speech changes		Confusion	
Tired or sleepy		Remembers the event	
Shaking / tremors		Feeling light-headed	
Problems communicating		Unsteady walking	
Loss of coordination (clumsy)		Change in appetite	
Digestive problems		Nausea / Vomiting	
Change in mood: depression, agitation, anger, irritability, excitability		Numbness (name part of body)	
Change in behaviour (detail in notes)		Headache	
Other:		Other:	
Other:		Other:	

Seizure Log

Date: Time: Duration:

Location:

Seizure Type:

If this was a cluster how many seizures?

Child's Mood:

What happened during the seizure?

What was happening around the time the seizure occurred?

Was there an Aura or warning? Yes ☐ No ☐ Describe:

Rescue medication if given:

VNS applied? Yes ☐ No ☐ Detail:

How long did it take your child to recover?

Notes:

Seizure Log

Possible Triggers			
High temperature		Illness or infection	
Missed or late medication		Temperature change	
Overtired		Missed or Poor Sleep	
Mood Change		Fast Breathing	
Missed Meal		Specific Food	
During Sleep		Upon Waking	
Time of day		Screen Use	
Low blood sugar		Low blood sodium	
OTC medications or supplements (please list)		Exercise (What did your child do?)	
Strong emotions - anxiety, stress, excitement, anger. Please describe:		Sensory - sounds, bright colours, flashing lights, patterns. Please describe:	
Other:		Other:	
Other:		Other:	

What happened after? (Recovery Period)			
Muscle weakness		Blurred or double vision	
Speech changes		Confusion	
Tired or sleepy		Remembers the event	
Shaking / tremors		Feeling light-headed	
Problems communicating		Unsteady walking	
Loss of coordination (clumsy)		Change in appetite	
Digestive problems		Nausea / Vomiting	
Change in mood: depression, agitation, anger, irritability, excitability		Numbness (name part of body)	
Change in behaviour (detail in notes)		Headache	
Other:		Other:	
Other:		Other:	

Seizure Log

Date: Time: Duration:

Location:

Seizure Type:

If this was a cluster how many seizures?

Child's Mood:

What happened during the seizure?

What was happening around the time the seizure occurred?

Was there an Aura or warning? Yes ☐ No ☐ Describe:

Rescue medication if given:

VNS applied? Yes ☐ No ☐ Detail:

How long did it take your child to recover?

Notes:

Seizure Log

Possible Triggers			
High temperature		Illness or infection	
Missed or late medication		Temperature change	
Overtired		Missed or Poor Sleep	
Mood Change		Fast Breathing	
Missed Meal		Specific Food	
During Sleep		Upon Waking	
Time of day		Screen Use	
Low blood sugar		Low blood sodium	
OTC medications or supplements (please list)		Exercise (What did your child do?)	
Strong emotions - anxiety, stress, excitement, anger. Please describe:		Sensory - sounds, bright colours, flashing lights, patterns. Please describe:	
Other:		Other:	
Other:		Other:	

What happened after? (Recovery Period)			
Muscle weakness		Blurred or double vision	
Speech changes		Confusion	
Tired or sleepy		Remembers the event	
Shaking / tremors		Feeling light-headed	
Problems communicating		Unsteady walking	
Loss of coordination (clumsy)		Change in appetite	
Digestive problems		Nausea / Vomiting	
Change in mood: depression, agitation, anger, irritability, excitability		Numbness (name part of body)	
Change in behaviour (detail in notes)		Headache	
Other:		Other:	
Other:		Other:	

Seizure Log

Date: Time: Duration:

Location:

Seizure Type:

If this was a cluster how many seizures?

Child's Mood:

What happened during the seizure?

What was happening around the time the seizure occurred?

Was there an Aura or warning? Yes ☐ No ☐ Describe:

Rescue medication if given:

VNS applied? Yes ☐ No ☐ Detail:

How long did it take your child to recover?

Notes:

Seizure Log

Possible Triggers	
High temperature	Illness or infection
Missed or late medication	Temperature change
Overtired	Missed or Poor Sleep
Mood Change	Fast Breathing
Missed Meal	Specific Food
During Sleep	Upon Waking
Time of day	Screen Use
Low blood sugar	Low blood sodium
OTC medications or supplements (please list)	Exercise (What did your child do?)
Strong emotions - anxiety, stress, excitement, anger. Please describe:	Sensory - sounds, bright colours, flashing lights, patterns. Please describe:
Other:	Other:
Other:	Other:

What happened after? (Recovery Period)	
Muscle weakness	Blurred or double vision
Speech changes	Confusion
Tired or sleepy	Remembers the event
Shaking / tremors	Feeling light-headed
Problems communicating	Unsteady walking
Loss of coordination (clumsy)	Change in appetite
Digestive problems	Nausea / Vomiting
Change in mood: depression, agitation, anger, irritability, excitability	Numbness (name part of body)
Change in behaviour (detail in notes)	Headache
Other:	Other:
Other:	Other:

Seizure Log

Date: _____ Time: _____ Duration: _____

Location: _____

Seizure Type: _____

If this was a cluster how many seizures? _____

Child's Mood: _____

What happened during the seizure? _____

_____

_____

_____

What was happening around the time the seizure occurred? _____

_____

_____

Was there an Aura or warning? Yes ☐ No ☐ Describe: _____

_____

Rescue medication if given: _____

VNS applied? Yes ☐ No ☐ Detail: _____

_____

How long did it take your child to recover? _____

Notes: _____

_____

_____

_____

Seizure Log

Possible Triggers			
High temperature		Illness or infection	
Missed or late medication		Temperature change	
Overtired		Missed or Poor Sleep	
Mood Change		Fast Breathing	
Missed Meal		Specific Food	
During Sleep		Upon Waking	
Time of day		Screen Use	
Low blood sugar		Low blood sodium	
OTC medications or supplements (please list)		Exercise (What did your child do?)	
Strong emotions - anxiety, stress, excitement, anger. Please describe:		Sensory - sounds, bright colours, flashing lights, patterns. Please describe:	
Other:		Other:	
Other:		Other:	

What happened after? (Recovery Period)			
Muscle weakness		Blurred or double vision	
Speech changes		Confusion	
Tired or sleepy		Remembers the event	
Shaking / tremors		Feeling light-headed	
Problems communicating		Unsteady walking	
Loss of coordination (clumsy)		Change in appetite	
Digestive problems		Nausea / Vomiting	
Change in mood: depression, agitation, anger, irritability, excitability		Numbness (name part of body)	
Change in behaviour (detail in notes)		Headache	
Other:		Other:	
Other:		Other:	

Seizure Log

Date: _____ Time: _____ Duration: _____

Location: _____

Seizure Type: _____

If this was a cluster how many seizures? _____

Child's Mood: _____

What happened during the seizure? _____

_____

_____

_____

What was happening around the time the seizure occurred? _____

_____

_____

Was there an Aura or warning? Yes ☐ No ☐ Describe: _____

_____

Rescue medication if given: _____

VNS applied? Yes ☐ No ☐ Detail: _____

How long did it take your child to recover? _____

Notes: _____

_____

_____

_____

Seizure Log

Possible Triggers			
High temperature		Illness or infection	
Missed or late medication		Temperature change	
Overtired		Missed or Poor Sleep	
Mood Change		Fast Breathing	
Missed Meal		Specific Food	
During Sleep		Upon Waking	
Time of day		Screen Use	
Low blood sugar		Low blood sodium	
OTC medications or supplements (please list)		Exercise (What did your child do?)	
Strong emotions - anxiety, stress, excitement, anger. Please describe:		Sensory - sounds, bright colours, flashing lights, patterns. Please describe:	
Other:		Other:	
Other:		Other:	

What happened after? (Recovery Period)			
Muscle weakness		Blurred or double vision	
Speech changes		Confusion	
Tired or sleepy		Remembers the event	
Shaking / tremors		Feeling light-headed	
Problems communicating		Unsteady walking	
Loss of coordination (clumsy)		Change in appetite	
Digestive problems		Nausea / Vomiting	
Change in mood: depression, agitation, anger, irritability, excitability		Numbness (name part of body)	
Change in behaviour (detail in notes)		Headache	
Other:		Other:	
Other:		Other:	

Seizure Log

Date: _____ Time: _____ Duration: _____

Location:

Seizure Type:

If this was a cluster how many seizures?

Child's Mood:

What happened during the seizure?

What was happening around the time the seizure occurred?

Was there an Aura or warning? Yes ☐ No ☐ Describe:

Rescue medication if given:

VNS applied? Yes ☐ No ☐ Detail:

How long did it take your child to recover?

Notes:

Seizure Log

Possible Triggers			
High temperature		Illness or infection	
Missed or late medication		Temperature change	
Overtired		Missed or Poor Sleep	
Mood Change		Fast Breathing	
Missed Meal		Specific Food	
During Sleep		Upon Waking	
Time of day		Screen Use	
Low blood sugar		Low blood sodium	
OTC medications or supplements (please list)		Exercise (What did your child do?)	
Strong emotions - anxiety, stress, excitement, anger. Please describe:		Sensory - sounds, bright colours, flashing lights, patterns. Please describe:	
Other:		Other:	
Other:		Other:	

What happened after? (Recovery Period)			
Muscle weakness		Blurred or double vision	
Speech changes		Confusion	
Tired or sleepy		Remembers the event	
Shaking / tremors		Feeling light-headed	
Problems communicating		Unsteady walking	
Loss of coordination (clumsy)		Change in appetite	
Digestive problems		Nausea / Vomiting	
Change in mood: depression, agitation, anger, irritability, excitability		Numbness (name part of body)	
Change in behaviour (detail in notes)		Headache	
Other:		Other:	
Other:		Other:	

Seizure Log

Date: _____ Time: _____ Duration: _____

Location: _____

Seizure Type: _____

If this was a cluster how many seizures? _____

Child's Mood: _____

What happened during the seizure? _____

_____

_____

_____

What was happening around the time the seizure occurred? _____

_____

_____

_____

Was there an Aura or warning? Yes ☐ No ☐ Describe: _____

_____

Rescue medication if given: _____

VNS applied? Yes ☐ No ☐ Detail: _____

How long did it take your child to recover? _____

Notes: _____

_____

_____

_____

Seizure Log

Possible Triggers			
High temperature		Illness or infection	
Missed or late medication		Temperature change	
Overtired		Missed or Poor Sleep	
Mood Change		Fast Breathing	
Missed Meal		Specific Food	
During Sleep		Upon Waking	
Time of day		Screen Use	
Low blood sugar		Low blood sodium	
OTC medications or supplements (please list)		Exercise (What did your child do?)	
Strong emotions - anxiety, stress, excitement, anger. Please describe:		Sensory - sounds, bright colours, flashing lights, patterns. Please describe:	
Other:		Other:	
Other:		Other:	

What happened after? (Recovery Period)			
Muscle weakness		Blurred or double vision	
Speech changes		Confusion	
Tired or sleepy		Remembers the event	
Shaking / tremors		Feeling light-headed	
Problems communicating		Unsteady walking	
Loss of coordination (clumsy)		Change in appetite	
Digestive problems		Nausea / Vomiting	
Change in mood: depression, agitation, anger, irritability, excitability		Numbness (name part of body)	
Change in behaviour (detail in notes)		Headache	
Other:		Other:	
Other:		Other:	

Seizure Log

Date: _____ Time: _____ Duration: _____

Location: _____

Seizure Type: _____

If this was a cluster how many seizures? _____

Child's Mood: _____

What happened during the seizure? _____

_____

_____

_____

What was happening around the time the seizure occurred? _____

_____

_____

Was there an Aura or warning? Yes ☐ No ☐ Describe: _____

_____

Rescue medication if given: _____

VNS applied? Yes ☐ No ☐ Detail: _____

How long did it take your child to recover? _____

Notes: _____

_____

_____

_____

Seizure Log

Possible Triggers			
High temperature		Illness or infection	
Missed or late medication		Temperature change	
Overtired		Missed or Poor Sleep	
Mood Change		Fast Breathing	
Missed Meal		Specific Food	
During Sleep		Upon Waking	
Time of day		Screen Use	
Low blood sugar		Low blood sodium	
OTC medications or supplements (please list)		Exercise (What did your child do?)	
Strong emotions - anxiety, stress, excitement, anger. Please describe:		Sensory - sounds, bright colours, flashing lights, patterns. Please describe:	
Other:		Other:	
Other:		Other:	

What happened after? (Recovery Period)			
Muscle weakness		Blurred or double vision	
Speech changes		Confusion	
Tired or sleepy		Remembers the event	
Shaking / tremors		Feeling light-headed	
Problems communicating		Unsteady walking	
Loss of coordination (clumsy)		Change in appetite	
Digestive problems		Nausea / Vomiting	
Change in mood: depression, agitation, anger, irritability, excitability		Numbness (name part of body)	
Change in behaviour (detail in notes)		Headache	
Other:		Other:	
Other:		Other:	

Seizure Log

Date: _____ Time: _____ Duration: _____

Location: _____

Seizure Type: _____

If this was a cluster how many seizures? _____

Child's Mood: _____

What happened during the seizure? _____
_____
_____
_____

What was happening around the time the seizure occurred? _____
_____
_____
_____

Was there an Aura or warning? Yes ☐ No ☐ Describe: _____
_____

Rescue medication if given: _____

VNS applied? Yes ☐ No ☐ Detail: _____

How long did it take your child to recover? _____

Notes: _____
_____
_____
_____

Seizure Log

Possible Triggers			
High temperature		Illness or infection	
Missed or late medication		Temperature change	
Overtired		Missed or Poor Sleep	
Mood Change		Fast Breathing	
Missed Meal		Specific Food	
During Sleep		Upon Waking	
Time of day		Screen Use	
Low blood sugar		Low blood sodium	
OTC medications or supplements (please list)		Exercise (What did your child do?)	
Strong emotions - anxiety, stress, excitement, anger. Please describe:		Sensory - sounds, bright colours, flashing lights, patterns. Please describe:	
Other:		Other:	
Other:		Other:	

What happened after? (Recovery Period)			
Muscle weakness		Blurred or double vision	
Speech changes		Confusion	
Tired or sleepy		Remembers the event	
Shaking / tremors		Feeling light-headed	
Problems communicating		Unsteady walking	
Loss of coordination (clumsy)		Change in appetite	
Digestive problems		Nausea / Vomiting	
Change in mood: depression, agitation, anger, irritability, excitability		Numbness (name part of body)	
Change in behaviour (detail in notes)		Headache	
Other:		Other:	
Other:		Other:	

Seizure Log

Date: _____ Time: _____ Duration: _____

Location: _____

Seizure Type: _____

If this was a cluster how many seizures? _____

Child's Mood: _____

What happened during the seizure? _____

What was happening around the time the seizure occurred? _____

Was there an Aura or warning? Yes ☐ No ☐ Describe: _____

Rescue medication if given: _____

VNS applied? Yes ☐ No ☐ Detail: _____

How long did it take your child to recover? _____

Notes: _____

Seizure Log

Possible Triggers

High temperature		Illness or infection	
Missed or late medication		Temperature change	
Overtired		Missed or Poor Sleep	
Mood Change		Fast Breathing	
Missed Meal		Specific Food	
During Sleep		Upon Waking	
Time of day		Screen Use	
Low blood sugar		Low blood sodium	
OTC medications or supplements (please list)		Exercise (What did your child do?)	
Strong emotions - anxiety, stress, excitement, anger. Please describe:		Sensory - sounds, bright colours, flashing lights, patterns. Please describe:	
Other:		Other:	
Other:		Other:	

What happened after? (Recovery Period)

Muscle weakness		Blurred or double vision	
Speech changes		Confusion	
Tired or sleepy		Remembers the event	
Shaking / tremors		Feeling light-headed	
Problems communicating		Unsteady walking	
Loss of coordination (clumsy)		Change in appetite	
Digestive problems		Nausea / Vomiting	
Change in mood: depression, agitation, anger, irritability, excitability		Numbness (name part of body)	
Change in behaviour (detail in notes)		Headache	
Other:		Other:	
Other:		Other:	

Seizure Log

Date: _____ Time: _____ Duration: _____

Location: _____

Seizure Type: _____

If this was a cluster how many seizures? _____

Child's Mood: _____

What happened during the seizure? _____

_____

_____

_____

What was happening around the time the seizure occurred? _____

_____

_____

Was there an Aura or warning? Yes ☐ No ☐ Describe: _____

_____

Rescue medication if given: _____

VNS applied? Yes ☐ No ☐ Detail: _____

How long did it take your child to recover? _____

Notes: _____

_____

_____

_____

Seizure Log

Possible Triggers			
High temperature		Illness or infection	
Missed or late medication		Temperature change	
Overtired		Missed or Poor Sleep	
Mood Change		Fast Breathing	
Missed Meal		Specific Food	
During Sleep		Upon Waking	
Time of day		Screen Use	
Low blood sugar		Low blood sodium	
OTC medications or supplements (please list)		Exercise (What did your child do?)	
Strong emotions - anxiety, stress, excitement, anger. Please describe:		Sensory - sounds, bright colours, flashing lights, patterns. Please describe:	
Other:		Other:	
Other:		Other:	

What happened after? (Recovery Period)			
Muscle weakness		Blurred or double vision	
Speech changes		Confusion	
Tired or sleepy		Remembers the event	
Shaking / tremors		Feeling light-headed	
Problems communicating		Unsteady walking	
Loss of coordination (clumsy)		Change in appetite	
Digestive problems		Nausea / Vomiting	
Change in mood: depression, agitation, anger, irritability, excitability		Numbness (name part of body)	
Change in behaviour (detail in notes)		Headache	
Other:		Other:	
Other:		Other:	

Seizure Log

Date: Time: Duration:

Location:

Seizure Type:

If this was a cluster how many seizures?

Child's Mood:

What happened during the seizure?

What was happening around the time the seizure occurred?

Was there an Aura or warning? Yes ☐ No ☐ Describe:

Rescue medication if given:

VNS applied? Yes ☐ No ☐ Detail:

How long did it take your child to recover?

Notes:

Seizure Log

Possible Triggers	
High temperature	Illness or infection
Missed or late medication	Temperature change
Overtired	Missed or Poor Sleep
Mood Change	Fast Breathing
Missed Meal	Specific Food
During Sleep	Upon Waking
Time of day	Screen Use
Low blood sugar	Low blood sodium
OTC medications or supplements (please list)	Exercise (What did your child do?)
Strong emotions - anxiety, stress, excitement, anger. Please describe:	Sensory - sounds, bright colours, flashing lights, patterns. Please describe:
Other:	Other:
Other:	Other:

What happened after? (Recovery Period)	
Muscle weakness	Blurred or double vision
Speech changes	Confusion
Tired or sleepy	Remembers the event
Shaking / tremors	Feeling light-headed
Problems communicating	Unsteady walking
Loss of coordination (clumsy)	Change in appetite
Digestive problems	Nausea / Vomiting
Change in mood: depression, agitation, anger, irritability, excitability	Numbness (name part of body)
Change in behaviour (detail in notes)	Headache
Other:	Other:
Other:	Other:

Seizure Log

Date: Time: Duration:

Location:

Seizure Type:

If this was a cluster how many seizures?

Child's Mood:

What happened during the seizure?

What was happening around the time the seizure occurred?

Was there an Aura or warning? Yes ☐ No ☐ Describe:

Rescue medication if given:

VNS applied? Yes ☐ No ☐ Detail:

How long did it take your child to recover?

Notes:

Seizure Log

Possible Triggers	
High temperature	Illness or infection
Missed or late medication	Temperature change
Overtired	Missed or Poor Sleep
Mood Change	Fast Breathing
Missed Meal	Specific Food
During Sleep	Upon Waking
Time of day	Screen Use
Low blood sugar	Low blood sodium
OTC medications or supplements (please list)	Exercise (What did your child do?)
Strong emotions - anxiety, stress, excitement, anger. Please describe:	Sensory - sounds, bright colours, flashing lights, patterns. Please describe:
Other:	Other:
Other:	Other:

What happened after? (Recovery Period)	
Muscle weakness	Blurred or double vision
Speech changes	Confusion
Tired or sleepy	Remembers the event
Shaking / tremors	Feeling light-headed
Problems communicating	Unsteady walking
Loss of coordination (clumsy)	Change in appetite
Digestive problems	Nausea / Vomiting
Change in mood: depression, agitation, anger, irritability, excitability	Numbness (name part of body)
Change in behaviour (detail in notes)	Headache
Other:	Other:
Other:	Other:

Seizure Log

Date: Time: Duration:

Location:

Seizure Type:

If this was a cluster how many seizures?

Child's Mood:

What happened during the seizure?

What was happening around the time the seizure occurred?

Was there an Aura or warning? Yes ☐ No ☐ Describe:

Rescue medication if given:

VNS applied? Yes ☐ No ☐ Detail:

How long did it take your child to recover?

Notes:

Seizure Log

Possible Triggers		
High temperature		Illness or infection
Missed or late medication		Temperature change
Overtired		Missed or Poor Sleep
Mood Change		Fast Breathing
Missed Meal		Specific Food
During Sleep		Upon Waking
Time of day		Screen Use
Low blood sugar		Low blood sodium
OTC medications or supplements (please list)		Exercise (What did your child do?)
Strong emotions - anxiety, stress, excitement, anger. Please describe:		Sensory - sounds, bright colours, flashing lights, patterns. Please describe:
Other:		Other:
Other:		Other:

What happened after? (Recovery Period)		
Muscle weakness		Blurred or double vision
Speech changes		Confusion
Tired or sleepy		Remembers the event
Shaking / tremors		Feeling light-headed
Problems communicating		Unsteady walking
Loss of coordination (clumsy)		Change in appetite
Digestive problems		Nausea / Vomiting
Change in mood: depression, agitation, anger, irritability, excitability		Numbness (name part of body)
Change in behaviour (detail in notes)		Headache
Other:		Other:
Other:		Other:

Seizure Log

Date: _____ Time: _____ Duration: _____

Location: _____

Seizure Type: _____

If this was a cluster how many seizures? _____

Child's Mood: _____

What happened during the seizure? _____

_____

_____

_____

What was happening around the time the seizure occurred? _____

_____

_____

_____

Was there an Aura or warning? Yes ☐ No ☐ Describe: _____

_____

Rescue medication if given: _____

VNS applied? Yes ☐ No ☐ Detail: _____

How long did it take your child to recover? _____

Notes: _____

_____

_____

_____

Seizure Log

Possible Triggers			
High temperature		Illness or infection	
Missed or late medication		Temperature change	
Overtired		Missed or Poor Sleep	
Mood Change		Fast Breathing	
Missed Meal		Specific Food	
During Sleep		Upon Waking	
Time of day		Screen Use	
Low blood sugar		Low blood sodium	
OTC medications or supplements (please list)		Exercise (What did your child do?)	
Strong emotions - anxiety, stress, excitement, anger. Please describe:		Sensory - sounds, bright colours, flashing lights, patterns. Please describe:	
Other:		Other:	
Other:		Other:	

What happened after? (Recovery Period)			
Muscle weakness		Blurred or double vision	
Speech changes		Confusion	
Tired or sleepy		Remembers the event	
Shaking / tremors		Feeling light-headed	
Problems communicating		Unsteady walking	
Loss of coordination (clumsy)		Change in appetite	
Digestive problems		Nausea / Vomiting	
Change in mood: depression, agitation, anger, irritability, excitability		Numbness (name part of body)	
Change in behaviour (detail in notes)		Headache	
Other:		Other:	
Other:		Other:	

Seizure Log

Date: Time: Duration:

Location:

Seizure Type:

If this was a cluster how many seizures?

Child's Mood:

What happened during the seizure?

What was happening around the time the seizure occurred?

Was there an Aura or warning? Yes ☐   No ☐   Describe:

Rescue medication if given:

VNS applied? Yes ☐ No ☐ Detail:

How long did it take your child to recover?

Notes:

Seizure Log

Possible Triggers			
High temperature		Illness or infection	
Missed or late medication		Temperature change	
Overtired		Missed or Poor Sleep	
Mood Change		Fast Breathing	
Missed Meal		Specific Food	
During Sleep		Upon Waking	
Time of day		Screen Use	
Low blood sugar		Low blood sodium	
OTC medications or supplements (please list)		Exercise (What did your child do?)	
Strong emotions - anxiety, stress, excitement, anger. Please describe:		Sensory - sounds, bright colours, flashing lights, patterns. Please describe:	
Other:		Other:	
Other:		Other:	

What happened after? (Recovery Period)			
Muscle weakness		Blurred or double vision	
Speech changes		Confusion	
Tired or sleepy		Remembers the event	
Shaking / tremors		Feeling light-headed	
Problems communicating		Unsteady walking	
Loss of coordination (clumsy)		Change in appetite	
Digestive problems		Nausea / Vomiting	
Change in mood: depression, agitation, anger, irritability, excitability		Numbness (name part of body)	
Change in behaviour (detail in notes)		Headache	
Other:		Other:	
Other:		Other:	

Seizure Log

Date: _____ Time: _____ Duration: _____

Location: _____

Seizure Type: _____

If this was a cluster how many seizures? _____

Child's Mood: _____

What happened during the seizure? _____

_____

_____

_____

What was happening around the time the seizure occurred? _____

_____

_____

Was there an Aura or warning? Yes ☐ No ☐ Describe: _____

_____

Rescue medication if given: _____

VNS applied? Yes ☐ No ☐ Detail: _____

How long did it take your child to recover? _____

Notes: _____

_____

_____

_____

Seizure Log

Possible Triggers			
High temperature		Illness or infection	
Missed or late medication		Temperature change	
Overtired		Missed or Poor Sleep	
Mood Change		Fast Breathing	
Missed Meal		Specific Food	
During Sleep		Upon Waking	
Time of day		Screen Use	
Low blood sugar		Low blood sodium	
OTC medications or supplements (please list)		Exercise (What did your child do?)	
Strong emotions - anxiety, stress, excitement, anger. Please describe:		Sensory - sounds, bright colours, flashing lights, patterns. Please describe:	
Other:		Other:	
Other:		Other:	

What happened after? (Recovery Period)			
Muscle weakness		Blurred or double vision	
Speech changes		Confusion	
Tired or sleepy		Remembers the event	
Shaking / tremors		Feeling light-headed	
Problems communicating		Unsteady walking	
Loss of coordination (clumsy)		Change in appetite	
Digestive problems		Nausea / Vomiting	
Change in mood: depression, agitation, anger, irritability, excitability		Numbness (name part of body)	
Change in behaviour (detail in notes)		Headache	
Other:		Other:	
Other:		Other:	